A MANUAL OF
Equine Diagnostic Procedures

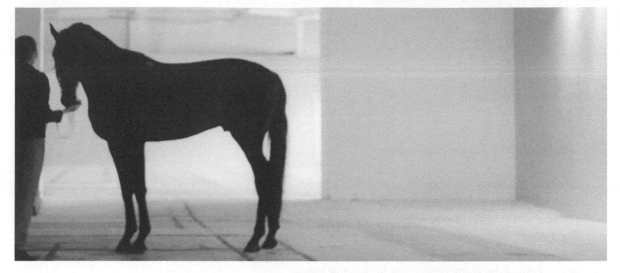

JOHN SCHUMACHER

DVM, MS, DIPLOMATE ACVIM

PROFESSOR OF LARGE ANIMAL MEDICINE AND SURGERY
COLLEGE OF VETERINARY MEDICINE
AUBURN UNIVERSITY
AUBURN, ALABAMA

H. DAVID MOLL

DVM, MS, DIPLOMATE ACVS

PROFESSOR OF EQUINE MEDICINE AND SURGERY
BIGGS-OXLEY CHAIR, EQUINE SPORTS MEDICINE
CENTER FOR VETERINARY HEALTH SCIENCES
OKLAHOMA STATE UNIVERSITY
STILLWATER, OKLAHOMA

Executive Editor: Carroll C. Cann
Development Editor: Susan L. Hunsberger
Creative Director: Sue Haun, 5640 Design www.fiftysixforty.com
Production Manager: Mike Albiniak, 5640 Design www.fiftysixforty.com

Teton NewMedia
P.O. Box 4833
Jackson, WY 83001

1-888-770-3165
tetonnewmedia.com

Library of Congress Cataloging-in-Publication Data

Moll, H. David.
    Manual of equine diagnostic procedures / H. David Moll, John Schumacher.
        p. cm.
    Includes bibliographical references and index.
    ISBN 1-893441-99-7 (alk. paper)
    1. Horses--Diseases--Diagnosis--Handbooks, manuals, etc. I. Title: Equine diagnostic
procedures. II. Schumacher, John (John R.) III. Title.

SF951.M65 2005
636.1'0896075--dc22

                                                            2005044043

TABLE OF CONTENTS

Chapters

DEDICATION

This book is dedicated to the memory of Dr. Joe Spano who was the heart and soul of the College of Veterinary Medicine, Auburn University. He was kind, wise and always ready to help.

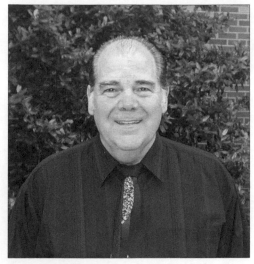

Dr. Joe Spano

ACKNOWLEDGEMENTS

We are grateful to many clinicians for their efforts to keep us from making errors in this book. We thank Drs. Frank Andrews, Todd Axlund, Kyle Braund, Gordon Brumbaugh, Bob Carson, Undine Christman, Paddy Dixon, Chris Dykstra, Pete Christopherson, Leanda Livesey, Charles Love, Kathy McGowan, Bill McMullan, John MacDonald, Leland Nuehring, Justin Perkins, David Pugh, David Ramsey, Dave Schmidt, Anne Schramme, Michael Schramme, Jim Schumacher, Steve Simpson, Joe Spano, Mary Beth Stanton, Allison Stewart, Jennifer Taintor, Dickson Varner, Betsy Welles, David Whitley, and Betsy Willis. If this book contains erroneous information, it is because these reviewers received an early draft and had no chance to examine later drafts for mistakes. Teri Hathcock, Joyce Stringfellow, Georgeann Ellis, and Elizabeth Whatley provided helpful technical advice, and Fred Lux's expertise of medical instrumentation was particularly helpful. It is hard to imagine that there is another editor out there who is as knowledgeable and easy to work with as Carroll Cann. One of the authors (JS), who spent some time in Harare, Zimbabwe, acknowledges the tutelage of Drs. John Barnwell and Karl van Loren. They are proof that expensive equipment or a myriad of drugs is not required to practice good equine medicine.

FORWARD

Very few diagnostic procedures require a great deal of expertise to perform. All the clinician needs is a good explanation and a chance to perform the procedure. Most procedures described in this book are easily performed and require little repetition for the clinician to become comfortable in their application. Veterinary academicians have an adage-- "see it once, do it once, then teach it." We hope that the procedures set forth in this book are described well enough that "see it once" can be replaced by "read it once."

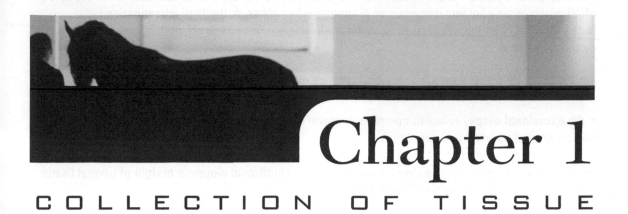

Chapter 1

COLLECTION OF TISSUE

Histological or cytological examination or microbial culture of tissue obtained from the living horse often provides an etiologic diagnosis or prognosis when other methods of investigation have failed. Biopsies can be categorized as excisional, incisional, aspirational, punch, and exfoliative cytology biopsies.

COLLECTION OF TISSUE

• An **excisional biopsy** refers to complete removal of a tissue for examination. Excisional biopsy can be both diagnostic and curative.

• When only a portion of the tissue in question is surgically removed, the biopsy is referred to as **incisional.** When performing either an excisional or an incisional biopsy, a margin of normal tissue should be removed, if possible. (Figure 1.1)

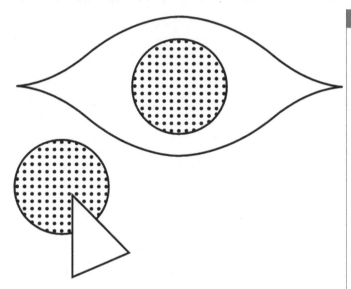

Figure 1.1

When performing either an excisional or an incisional biopsy, a margin of normal tissue should also be removed, if possible.

• **Needle aspiration biopsies** are taken with a hypodermic needle attached to a syringe. The firmer the tissue, the larger the syringe that should be used. When in doubt, a 12mL syringe is usually adequate. Use of 18- to 25- ga (1.2- to 0.5- mm) needles is recommended. Needles larger than 21-ga (0.8mm) however, tend to collect tissue cores rather than free cells for cytology, and may result in rupture of cells. The site of puncture is surgically prepared. To avoid contaminating the biopsy with cutaneous debris, a stab incision is made in the skin before inserting the needle or, alternatively, a styleted needle is pushed through skin and then the stylet is removed (Figure 1.2). Or by using a Menghini Soft Tissue Aspiration Needle (Popper & Sons, Inc. 300 Denton Ave., New Hyde Park, NY 11040 USA) (Figure 1.3), contamination of the biopsy with cutaneous debris is avoided. The needle is then advanced into the lesion. Once the needle is within the lesion, the syringe plunger is pulled back to create negative pressure. *Even if fluid or tissue is not seen in the syringe or needle hub, the needle shaft may contain enough cells for diagnosis.* Before the needle is removed from the lesion, negative pressure should be released slowly. The needle should be redirected in several different planes, and the procedure repeated. After removing the needle from tissue, the syringe is disconnected from the needle, filled with air, the needle is replaced, and the plunger is rapidly depressed to blow cells onto a microscope slide. Another microscope slide is placed over this slide, and then the two slides are separated by pulling the slides apart in a horizontal plane to create a thin layer of cells for microscopic examination.

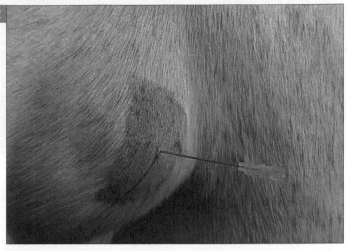

Figure 1.2

To avoid contaminating the biopsy with cutaneous debris, a stab incision is made in the skin before inserting the needle or, alternatively, a styleted needle is pushed through skin and then the stylet is removed.

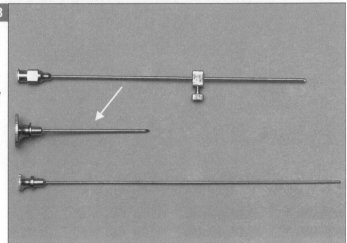

Figure 1.3

A Menghini Soft Tissue Biopsy Needle prevents contamination of the biopsy with cutaneous debris. The sharp pointed trochar (arrow) is used for the initial skin pierce.

- **Needle punch biopsies** are obtained using specialized cutting needles designed to remove a core of tissue. Examples include the:
  » **Tru-Cut style needle,** which is used to biopsy any solid lesion or organ. These needles are available as manually operated or spring-loaded, automated instruments (Figures. 1.4 & 1.5). The Tru-Cut is a double needle consisting of a hollow outer needle called the *cannula* and an inner needle called the *stylet.* To place the needle properly, the *cannula* is advanced to the site of interest, not *into* the site (Figure 1.6).
  » **Menghini** (Figure 1.3) **and Vim Silverman** (Figure 1.7) **needles,** which are designed for liver, kidney and soft tissue biopsy.
  » **Jamshidi-type needle,** which is designed for bone marrow biopsy or aspiration (Figures 1.8, 6.1).
  » **Bergstrom-type biopsy needle,** which is used to sample muscle (Figures 1.9, 23.2).

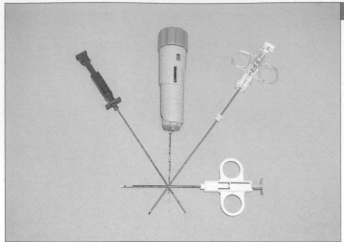

Figure 1.4

Tru-Cut style biopsy needles are available as manually operated or spring-loaded, automated instruments.

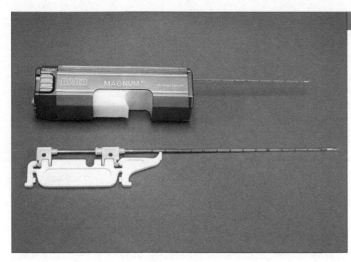

Figure 1.5

The Bard Magnum® biopsy instrument (C.R. Bard, Inc., Covington, GA. 30014) uses disposable needles that are available in different gauges and lengths.

CORRECT PLACEMENT OF BIOPSY NEEDLE

INCORRECT PLACEMENT OF BIOPSY NEEDLE

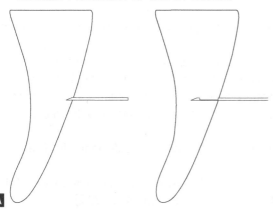

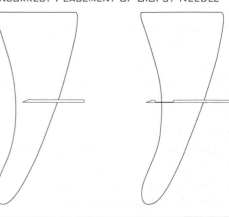

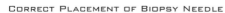

Figure 1.6A & B   *The Tru-Cut is a double needle consisting of a hollow outer needle called the cannula and an inner needle called the stylet. To place the Tru-cut needle properly, the cannula is advanced to the site of interest **(A)**, not into the site **(B)**.*

Figure 1.7

The Vim Silverman needle is designed for liver, kidney and soft tissue biopsy.

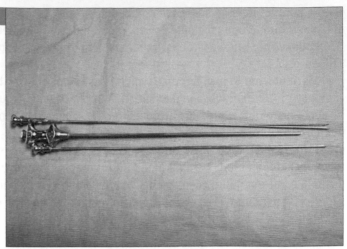

Figure 1.8

The Jamshidi-type needle is designed for bone marrow biopsy or aspiration.

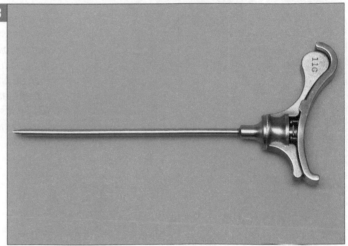

Figure 1.9

The Bergstrom-type biopsy needle is used to sample muscle. Shown is the U. C. H. Skeletal Muscle Biopsy Needle (Popper & Sons, Inc. 300 Denton Ave., New Hyde Park, NY 11040 USA).

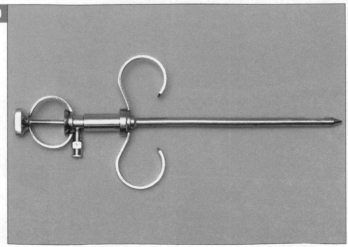

- **Jaw punch biopsies** are obtained using instruments with alligator-like jaws that remove a portion of tissue that includes the outer surface of the tissue sampled. Examples include the:
  - » **Endoscopic biopsy forceps,** which seldom obtains enough tissue for accurate interpretation (Figure 13.4).
  - » **Mare uterine biopsy forceps,** which is used not only for biopsy of endometrium, but also for biopsy of rectal mucosa and tissue in the nasal cavity (Figures 1.10, 17.1).

To avoid histological artifacts, tissue should be removed from biopsy needles with a hypodermic needle rather than by using fingers (Figure 1.11).

- **Exfoliative cytology** refers to study of cells obtained from skin, mucosa, internal organs, or body cavities. Exfoliated cells are obtained by 1) scraping tissue, 2) pressing a microscope slide against tissue (i.e., direct impression smear), 3) pressing a swab against a lesion, and then to a microscope slide (i.e., an indirect impression smear). Moistening a swab with saline before a smear is obtained indirectly may improve the quality of the smear.

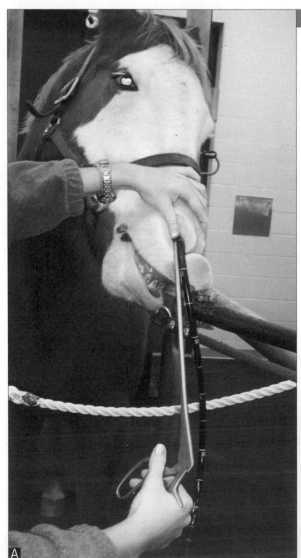

Figure 1.10A & B

By using a mare endometrial biopsy forceps for endoscopic guided biopsy of nasal tumors (A) rather than an endoscopic biopsy forceps, adequate tissue (B) for histological diagnosis is more likely to be obtained.

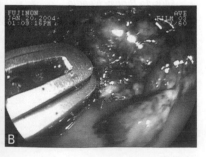

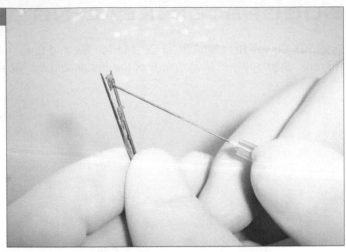

Figure 1.11

To avoid histological artifacts, tissue should be removed from biopsy needles with a hypodermic needle rather than by using fingers.

HANDLING OF SPECIMENS FOR HISTOLOGICAL EXAMINATION

- Cores of tissue can be removed from the biopsy needle with forceps, a hypodermic needle, or by agitation of the biopsy needle in fixative (or a transport medium).
- Impression smears for cytological examination can be made before the tissue is submitted for histological examination (although this may decrease the quality of the specimen for histological examination) (Figure 1.12).
- Tissue can be placed in a commercially available transport medium for culture. Alternatively, tissue for culture can be transported in sterile, physiological saline solution for up to 24 hours.
- Tissue is placed in a fixative. Rule of thumb: **use 10-15 volumes of fixative to one volume of tissue.**
- **10% formalin** is the most commonly used fixative. Neutral buffered formalin is preferred over plain formalin.
- **Bouin's solution** is often used to fix intestinal mucosa, endometrium, and endocrine tissue. It provides excellent preservation of cellular detail, but tissue fixed in this solution for over 24 hours becomes brittle and difficult to section. When delay of tissue processing is anticipated, tissue can be allowed to fix in Bouin's solution (for at least 2 hours and no longer than 24 hours) and then transferred to 70% ethyl alcohol or formalin.
- **3 or 4% buffered gluteraldehyde** (made from a refrigerated 25% stock solution just before use) is used to fix tissue for electron microscopy.

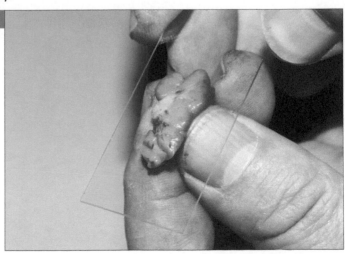

Figure 1.12

Impression smears for cytological examination can be made before the tissue is submitted for histological examination.

SUGGESTED READING

Tyler RD, Cowell RL, MacAllister CG, Morton RJ, and Caruso KJ. Introduction. In: Cowell RL, Tyler RD, eds. *Cytology and Hematology of the Horse. 2nd ed.* Mosby: Philadelphia; 2002; 1-18.

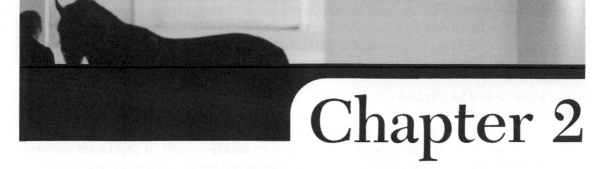

Chapter 2

HANDLING OF FLUID SPECIMENS

HANDLING OF FLUID SPECIMENS

- Samples of fluid should be submitted to a laboratory within 12 hours for processing
- **or,** fluid can be mixed with an equal volume of **40% or 50% ethanol** (100-proof vodka is 50% ethanol) (or other fixatives recommended by the laboratory). Special stains are required for cytological evaluation of cells from fluid mixed with ethanol and *morphology of cells fixed with ethanol is difficult to interpret.*
- or, a smear should be prepared

   a) **for samples with low viscosity:** If the specimen is highly cellular, a routine hematologic spread technique is used. A drop of fluid is placed on one end of a slide, and then another slide (spreader slide) is backed into it. The spreader slide is then pushed ***rapidly*** forward (at about a 45° angle) to create a film (Figure 2.1). The edges of the film must remain on the slide. If the specimen is not highly cellular, it should be spun at 1500 rpm, and the supernatant gently decanted. Remove nearly all the supernatant, leaving a volume of fluid approximately equal to the volume of sediment. The last drop of fluid is agitated and used to make the smear.

   b) **for samples with high viscosity (i.e., synovial fluid):** The spreader slide is pushed ***slowly*** forward to create a film, or the spreader slide is held at a greater angle (25°) (Figure 2.1). A *squash preparation* is another method used successfully to make smears of viscous samples. A drop of fluid or mucus is placed on one slide and another slide is laid flat on top, overlapping about 3/4 of the bottom slide. The two slides are pulled apart in horizontal planes while the fluid is still spreading between them (Figure 2.2).

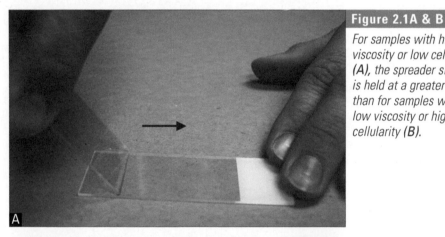

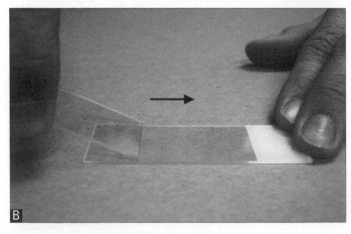

Figure 2.1A & B

For samples with high viscosity or low cellularity (A), the spreader slide is held at a greater angle than for samples with low viscosity or high cellularity (B).

A

B

c) **for samples that contain tissue fragments (i.e., bone marrow):** a large drop of fluid is placed at one end of a slide, and excess fluid or blood is aspirated back into the syringe leaving behind heavier particles of tissue. Then blood-film type smear or squash preparation can be made (Figure 6.4).

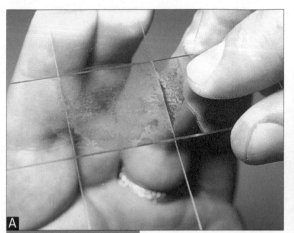 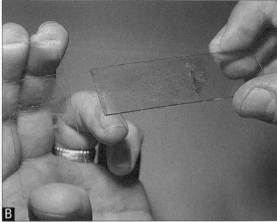

Figure 2.2A & B *A squash preparation can be made by placing a slide on top of the one with the sample (A) and then pulling the slides apart in a horizontal direction (B).*

FIXATION OF SMEARS

a) When smears are to be stained with Romanowsky-type stains (e.g., Wright's stain, Giemsa's stain, or Diff Quik) slides should be air-dried. A slide can be rapidly *air-dried* by waving it in the air or by holding it in front of a fan or a hair drier set on low.

b) Smears that are to be stained with Papanicolaou stain should be fixed before they dry (i.e., *wet fixation*). For this purpose, commercial fixatives can be used to spray the smear while it is still wet. Hair spray is also often suitable to wet fix slides for special stains. Hair spray that contains no perfume or lanolin (i.e., the cheaper brands) should be used. Because wet-fixed smears are not suitable for staining with Romanowsky-type stains, which are most commonly used, few veterinary cytologists use wet-fixed smears and Papanicolaou staining. The method of fixation preferred by the laboratory to which slides are sent should be determined.

SUGGESTED READING

Tyler RD, Cowell RL, MacAllister CG, Morton RJ, and Caruso KJ. Introduction. In: Cowell RL, Tyler RD, eds. *Cytology and Hematology of the Horse. 2nd ed.* Mosby: Philadelphia; 2002, 1-18.

Chapter 3

HANDLING OF SPECIMENS FOR BACTERIAL CULTURE AND VIRAL ISOLATION

Table 3.1
Handling of Specimens for Bacterial Culture and Viral Isolation

Aerobic/Fungal Specimen	Suggested Transport Device	Storage or Transport
Abscess/wound (aerobic)	Port-A-Cul tube or vial*	Refrigerate/cold pack
Blood Culture	Blood culture bottle (Columbia Broth, Trypticase Soy Broth, or Supplemented Peptone Broth)* (1:10 ratio of blood to media)	Room Temperature
Catheter (distal 2 inches)	Sterile specimen cup	Refrigerate (add a few drops of sterile physiologic saline solution to keep moist) cold pack
Eye (swab specimen)	Swab with transport medium (e.g., Amies or Stuart's medium)	Refrigerate/cold pack
Eye (corneal specimen)	Tissue placed in sterile physiological saline solution	Room Temperature
Feces	Screw-cap specimen cup (clean); Preserved w/ Cary Blair transport medium*	Refrigerate/cold pack
Fluids (CSF, pleural, etc.)	Port-A-Cul vial* or sterile tube	Room Temperature
Fluids (pericardial)	Port-A-Cul vial* or sterile tube	Refrigerate/cold pack
Hair, scale, crust	Paper envelope	Room Temperature
Milk	Sterile tube	Refrigerate/cold pack
Endometrial swab	Port-A-Cul tube or vial*, or swab placed in a transport medium (e.g. Amies or Stuart's medium)	Refrigerate/cold pack
Respiratory secretions (TTW, BAL)	Port-A-Cul vial* or sterile tube	Refrigerate/cold pack
Tissue (biopsy)	Port-A-Cul vial *or sterile tube w/ sterile physiological saline solution	Room Temperature
Urine	Sterile tube	Refrigerate/cold pack

Table 3.1 Continued

Anaerobic Specimen	Suggested Transport Device	Storage or Transport
Abscess/wound	Port-A-Cul tube or vial*	Room Temperature
Fluids	Port-A-Cul vial*	Room Temperature
Tissues/swabs	Port-A-Cul tube*	Room Temperature
Viral Specimen		
Tissues/swabs	Place samples separately in plastic food storage bags	< 48hr to lab -cool to 4° C and ship on ice packs > 48 hr to lab –freeze to -17° C (household freezer) and ship on ice packs

(Source: Manual of Clinical Microbiology, 7th ed. Murray, PR, ed. ASM Press, Washington, D. C., 1999.)
*BBL Microbiological Systems, Becton, Dickinson and Co., Sparks, MD 21152

Sufficient specimen must be submitted for each test requested. To process for aerobic, anaerobic, and fungal culture, three swabs or sufficient specimen to be divided between three different media should be submitted.

Fluid specimens should be submitted in a **Port-A-Cul *vial*** (flip top with rubber stopper) (Figure 3.1). Expel all air from syringe and using a new needle, layer fluid on top of transport medium (to minimize oxygen concentration within the vial).

Tissue specimens should be submitted in a **Port-A-Cul *tube*** (screw-cap tube) (Figure 3.1). Push the specimen to the *bottom* of the tube. For a specimen too large for the Port-A-Cul tube, tissue is placed in a sterile specimen container with a *small* amount of sterile physiologic saline solution to prevent desiccation. If anaerobic culture is needed, remove a small portion of tissue and place it near the bottom of an additional Port-A-Cul tube.

Swab specimens should be submitted in a **Port-A-Cul *tube*** or similar culturette device if only aerobic bacterial culture is needed.

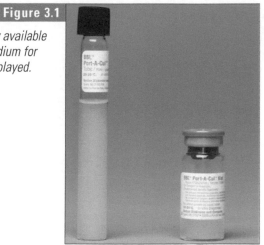

Figure 3.1

Commercially available transport medium for culture is displayed.

Chapter 4

COLLECTION OF HAIR, CRUSTS, AND SKIN

SKIN SCRAPINGS

Skin scrapings in the horse are primarily of value for the diagnosis of microscopic ectoparasitism. Surface and burrowing mites, and some nematode larva can be identified during examination of skin scrapings. Because ectoparasitism in the horse is uncommon, and often identified by alternative methods, skin scrapings are often omitted from the routine dermatological examination.

Indications
• For investigation of pruritic skin disease typical of a parasitic infestation. Pruritic skin disease of the limb should be investigated with skin scrapings, because chorioptic mange is occasionally a cause of skin disease involving the distal portion of the limbs of horses.
• Many equine dermatologists consider skin scrapings to be part of a routine dermatological examination.

Materials
• Hair clippers (optional)
• #10 or 22 scalpel blade to decrease the chance of lacerating the skin, the blade should be dulled before use. Alternatively, a bone curette can be used for scraping (Figure 4.1).
• Glass microscope slides, coverslips and a container for transport of the slides
• Mineral oil, to immobilize mange mites making them easier to identify, an insecticide can be added to the mineral oil to further immobilize mites.

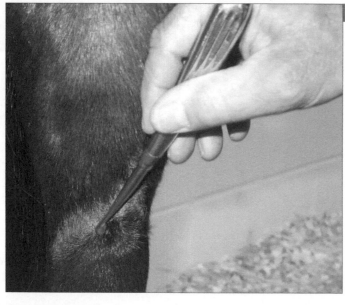

Figure 4.1

A bone curette can be used to collect a skin scraping.

Procedure
• A site at the periphery of an unexcoriated lesion is selected.
• Hair that may interfere with the scraping can be removed with a clipper.
• Mineral oil is applied to the area of skin selected for scraping.
• The scalpel blade is held perpendicular to the surface of the skin and a large area is superficially scraped. Then a smaller area of skin within the scraped area is scraped until capillary bleeding is observed. Squeezing the skin prior to, and during deep scraping may improve collection of parasites.
• The tissue collected is transferred to a glass slide and a cover slip is applied, or alternatively, transferred to a container for transport.

- Samples should be examined as soon as possible to avoid distortion or escape of collected parasites. At least five samples should be examined before a negative diagnosis can be made with any confidence.
- To increase diagnostic effectiveness, material from a scraping can be added to a saturated salt solution for flotation or centrifugation. Mites and ova, which rise to the top of the solution, can be found by microscopic examination of several drops of the surface solution.

COLLECTION OF HAIR AND CRUSTS FOR DERMATOPHYTE CULTURE

Diagnosis of dermatophytosis is best confirmed by fungal culture of hair, scales or crusts. Direct microscopic examination of hair, scales or crusts from affected and adjacent skin may reveal microorganisms. Because dematophytes that commonly affect horses do not fluoresce, a Wood's lamp examination is not a reliable method of diagnosis.

Indications

Any focal or generalized expanding area of alopecia should be examined for dermatophytes especially if the lesions involve the head, neck, saddle or girth areas, or limbs of horses, especially young horses. Dermatophyte lesions often contain scales or crusts and may or may not be pruritic.

Materials

- Clean hemostats
- An envelope for collection of hair and crusts
- A clearing agent such as 10 to 20% solution of potassium hydroxide (KOH) (Remel, Inc. 12076 Sante Fe Drive, Lenexa, KS 66215). Clearing agents digest hair and debris so that fungal elements can be seen more clearly. For identifying equine dermatophytes, using a clearing agent is not essential.
- A light microscope and microscope slides and coverslips
- 70% Isopropyl alcohol or a non-antiseptic soap
- Dermatophyte testing medium (DTM) (Sab-Duets plates, Bacti-Labs, Mountain View, CA; Derma Tube, Remel, Inc. 12076 Sante Fe Drive, Lenexa, KS 66215; or Dermatophyte Test Medium, Blue Ridge Biologicals, Inc. Box 634 Hickory, NC 28603) (Figure 4.2)

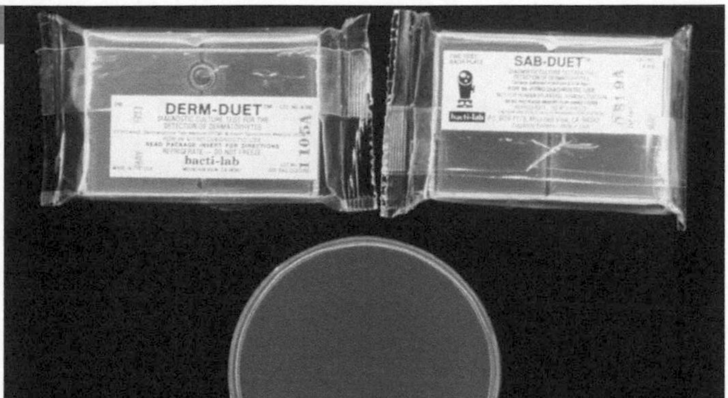

Figure 4.2

Dermatophyte testing medium.

EXAMINATION FOR DERMATOPHYTES

Procedure

• The lesion can be wiped with alcohol or washed with a non-antiseptic soap to decrease the growth of contaminants before hairs are collected for culture. *The lesion should be dry when the specimen is collected* (to decrease growth of contaminants).

• Using a clean hemostat, broken hairs from the *periphery of the lesion* are plucked in the direction of growth. Several lesions should be sampled to increase the likelihood of isolating a dermatophyte.

• **For direct microscopic examination,** hair and crusts are suspended in a clearing solution. If a clearing solution is unavailable, samples can be viewed in mineral oil or water. Hair and crusts are examined for hyphae and arthroconidia, using the 10 and 40x objective of the microscope. Clinicians inexperienced at direct examination of hair for identification of dermatophytes should submit specimens to a laboratory with experienced personnel.

• **For inoculation of DTM,** clumps of hair should be teased apart and a few affected hairs are gently pressed onto the medium. Avoid penetrating the surface of the medium with the samples. Innoculation of the dermatophyte-testing medium with an excessive amount of hair may result in over-growth of contaminants.

• When using DTM in a vial, the cap of the vial should not be tightened because fungi require oxygen for growth. Innoculated samples should be incubated at room temperature (for growth of *Trichophyton equinum, Microsporum canis,* or *Microsporum gypseum*) and at 37°C (for growth of *Trichophyton verrucosum*).

• Identification of dermatophyte colonies is aided by microscopic examination (10X). A slide can be prepared by touching the colony with transparent cellophane tape and then applying the tape to a microscope slide to which a drop of water or lactophenol cotton blue has been added.

Interpretation

• Even experienced technicians often fail to identify dermatophytes during direct examination of infected hair. Hairs infected with dermatophytes are often fragmented, pale or swollen. Fungal spores are very small, round to oval, and often grouped as chains along the hair shaft (Figure 4.3).

• Dermatophyte colonies grow in approximately three to 14 days. Prior treatment of the horse with antifungal agents may delay growth of dermatophytes. Cultures from treated horses should be incubated for 21 days.

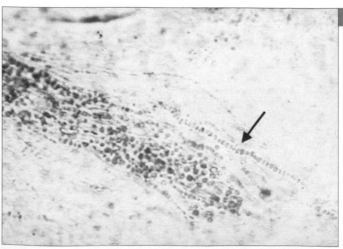

Figure 4.3

Dermatophytes are rarely identified, even by experienced technicians during direct examination of infected hair.

- Dermatophytes grow as white-, beige-, or cream-colored colonies. Contaminant colonies are often black, green, gray or brown.
- Growth of dermatophytes causes a rise in pH, which causes the medium to change from yellow to red around the area of colony growth. The color changes simultaneously with colony growth (Figure 4.4). Contaminants may also cause a red-color change in the medium, but the change is usually delayed and does not occur simultaneously with colony growth (Figure 4.5). *To correctly interpret test results, the samples must be examined daily.*
- Identification of dermatophytes requires microscopic examination of the colonies grown on DTM. Most *Microsporum* species can be identified by recognizing characteristic macroconidia spores. Speciation of *Trychophyton* species requires additional testing that involves determining specific growth requirements. Most microbiology texts include information concerning dermatophyte identification.

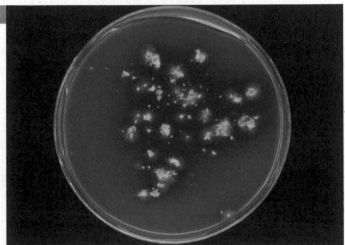

Figure 4.4

Dermatophytes cause the medium to change from yellow to red around the area of colony growth. The color change is simultaneous with colony growth.

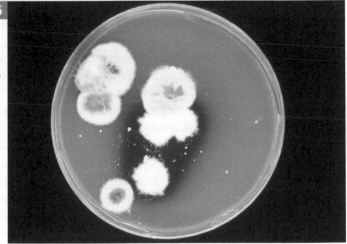

Figure 4.5

Contaminants may also cause a red-color change in the medium, but the change is usually delayed and not simultaneous with colony growth.

SKIN BIOPSY

Skin biopsies are most helpful in the diagnosis of nodular skin disease. Some diffuse skin diseases cannot be diagnosed without histological examination of affected skin. A skin biopsy taken early from an untraumatized site is much more valuable than a biopsy from a chronic lesion. Multiple skin biopsies increase the chance for an accurate diagnosis.

Indications

- Suspected neoplastic lesions
- Nonhealing ulcers
- Any dermatosis not responding as expected to treatment
- Any dermatosis with an unusual appearance
- Definitive diagnosis of skin disease for which treatment will be expensive, dangerous, or time consuming

Contraindications

- None, although the location of the lesion may influence the type of biopsy taken. For example, an excisional or incisional biopsy (see Figure 1.1) of a lesion on the back of a riding horse may be contraindicated, unless results of a less invasive biopsy technique (i.e., a needle or aspiration biopsy) indicate that an incisional biopsy is necessary for diagnosis or that excision is necessary for resolution of the lesion.
- Incisional biopsy of a sarcoid may initiate aggressive growth of the tumor.
- Sites over vessels, joints, and bony prominences are best avoided.

Materials

- Local anesthetic solution, syringe, and a 20- to 25-ga (0.9- to 0.5-mm) needle
- A 4- to 10-mm skin biopsy punch (i.e., AcuPunch Biopsy Punch, Acuderm Inc., Ft. Lauderdale, FL 33309) **Or**
- A scalpel blade, thumb forceps, needle holders, suture material (or staples), and a tongue depressor or cardboard
- Fixative (usually 10% formalin)

Procedure

- Skin should be minimally prepared so that superficial lesions are not removed during preparation. Hair can be clipped, and the site rinsed with alcohol, but *skin should not be shaved or scrubbed. Use of iodine prep may interfere with staining.*
- Regional anesthesia with a local anesthetic agent is ideal, when possible (e.g., limbs or the perineal region), or local anesthetic agent can be injected subcutaneously directly under the site of biopsy or injected around the lesion as a ring block.
- A circular piece of skin and subcutaneous tissue can be removed by continuous circular motion (in one direction only) of a skin biopsy punch (Figure 4.6). Most pathologists prefer samples >6mm. For deep lesions, the biopsy punch can be reinserted into a site to remove more tissue **Or**
- Using a scalpel blade, an elliptical piece of skin and subcutaneous tissue that contains both grossly normal and abnormal skin can be removed. *Biopsies of ulcerative lesions should always include an edge of normal epithelium. Vesicular and bullous lesions should be biopsied in their entirety.*
- After the skin is cut with a punch or scalpel blade, the subcutaneous tissue and the skin is grasped and lifted *delicately* with a forceps (alternatively, the biopsy specimen is held and lifted with a small gauge needle pushed through an edge of the specimen) and cut free with a scalpel blade. Some pathologists emphasize that, to avoid artifactual histopathogical changes, the biopsy specimen not be freed with a scissors. Excess blood should be removed from the sample by blotting with a gauze sponge prior to fixing.
- Touch preps for cytological evaluation can be made at this time by gently rolling and pressing the sample against a microscope slide.

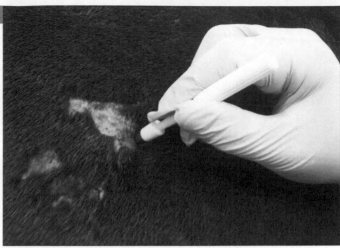

Figure 4.6

A circular piece of diseased skin surrounding normal skin and subcutaneous tissue, can be removed by continuous circular motion of an AcuPunch skin biopsy punch.

• Elliptical biopsies should be mounted so they don't curl during fixation. The subcutaneous side of the specimen is placed on a tongue depressor or piece of cardboard and gently pressed so that it adheres to the surface.

• 10% formalin is the usual fixative for skin. Bouin's solution is also suitable, but only for small or thin biopsies because it poorly penetrates tissue. Skin should not be stored in Bouin's solution for over 24 hours. Michel's fixative is sometimes used to fix skin for immunoflorescence studies when immune-mediated skin disease is suspected, but formalin-fixed skin may also be suitable for diagnosis of immune-mediated skin disease. When in doubt concerning fixation of tissue, the pathologist should be consulted before biopsies are taken.

• Elliptical biopsy sites are closed with sutures or staples. Punch biopsy sites are often closed with a single suture or staple or are left to heal as an open wound.

Interpretation

A pathologist with knowledge of equine skin disease should interpret samples submitted for histological examination. To aid in interpretation, a history, description of physical findings, and suspected diagnosis should always accompany the specimen.

SUGGESTED READINGS

Evans AG, Stannard AA. Diagnostic approach to equine skin disease. *Compendium on Continuing Education for the Practicing Veterinarian.* 8:652-660, 1986.

Pascoe RRR, Knottenbelt DC. *Manual of Equine Dermatology.* New York: WB Saunders Co; 1999:21-34.

Kowalski JJ. Bacterial and mycotic infections. In: Reed SM and Bayly WM, eds. *Equine Internal Medicine.* Philadelphia: WB Saunders Co; 1998:61-93.

Scott DW, Miller WH. Jr. *Equine Dermatology.* St. Louis: Elsevier Science; 2003:59-162.

COLLECTION OF BLOOD FROM

Chapter 5

COLLECTION OF BLOOD FROM SITES OTHER THAN A JUGULAR VEIN

COLLECTION OF BLOOD FROM SITES OTHER THAN A JUGULAR VEIN

Although blood of horses is usually collected from a jugular vein, alternate veins for collecting blood include the transverse facial vein, cephalic vein, and the lateral thoracic vein (Figures 5.1 & 5.2).

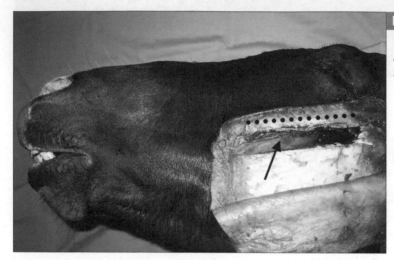

Figure 5.1

The transverse facial vein is located below the facial crest (dotted line).

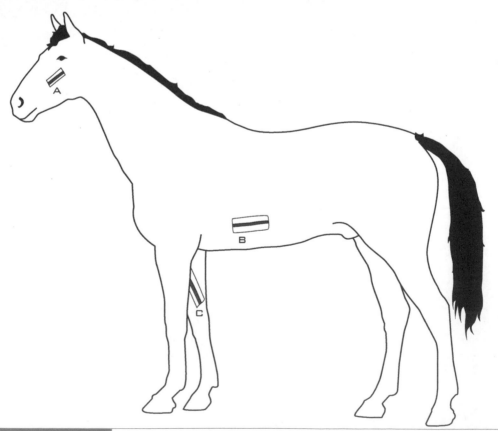

Figure 5.2   *Alternate veins for collecting blood include the transverse facial vein (A), cephalic vein (B), and the lateral thoracic vein (C).*

Some horses have prominent lateral thoracic veins, especially draft horses (Figure 5.3), but for many horses this vein is difficult to find. Blood can be safely collected from the saphenous vein in recumbent foals or anesthetized horses.

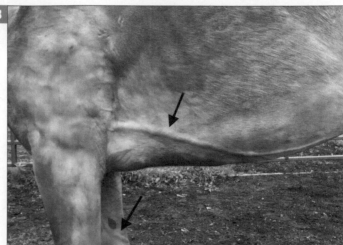

Figure 5.3

The lateral thoracic vein and cephalic vein (arrows) are prominent on this Belgium mare, but for some horses, the lateral thoracic vein is difficult to find.

Indications
- To collect blood from horses with thrombosis of one or both jugular veins
- To avoid excessive venipuncture of the jugular veins of horses prone to venous thrombosis (e.g., horses with colitis)

Materials
- Alcohol and cotton for site preparation
- When only a packed cell volume (PCV) is needed, materials include a 25-ga, 5/8- in (0.5 x 16 mm) needle, sealing clay, and a heparinized microhematocrit tube.
- When larger quantities of blood are needed, materials include a 20-ga x 1.5-in (0.9- x 38-mm) needle, a 10- or 20-mL syringe, and EDTA and plain glass tubes. Blood can also be collected directly into blood collection tubes using a blood collection needle.

COLLECTION OF BLOOD FROM THE TRANSVERSE FACIAL VEIN

Procedure
- A needle is inserted through skin, below the facial crest, on or rostral to a line perpendicular to the facial crest drawn from the medial canthus of the eye. To obtain only enough blood for a PCV, a small gauge needle such as a 25-ga, 5/8-in (0.5- x 16-mm) needle is inserted until the hub fills with blood. Then, the end of a microhematocrit tube is placed into the needle hub and allowed to fill by capillary action (Figure 5.4). **Or:**

• A 20-ga needle with a syringe attached is inserted below the facial crest near a line perpendicular to the facial crest drawn from the medial canthus of the eye until the point of the needle strikes bone, the plunger of the syringe is gently retracted, as the needle is slowly withdrawn, until the syringe begins to fill with blood (Figure 5.5).

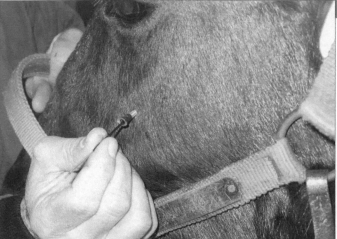

Figure 5.4

To collect a small amount of blood from the transverse facial vein, a needle is inserted through skin, just below the facial crest, on a line perpendicular to the facial crest drawn from the medial canthus of the eye.

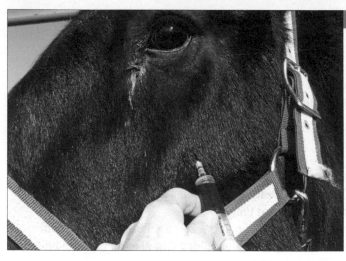

Figure 5.5

To collect a large amount of blood from the transverse facial vein, 20-ga, 1.5 in needle with a syringe attached is inserted below the facial crest until the point of the needle strikes bone. The plunger of the syringe is gently retracted, as the needle is slowly withdrawn, until the syringe begins to fill with blood.

Complications

• Some horses become head shy after the procedure has been performed numerous times.
• Hair loss over the site of venipuncture may occur, possibly from skin irritation from repeated application of alcohol.
• A transient hematoma at the venipuncture site (rare)
• Facial nerve paresis has been reported, but placement of the needle distal to the recommended site of venipuncture was the suspected cause. The facial nerve lies about 2-cm below the recommended site of venipuncture.

SUGGESTED READING

Sweeney CR, Parente E. Alternate site for venipuncture in the horse: The transverse facial vein. *Proceedings, Annual Convention of the American Association of Equine Practitioners,* 41:272-273, 1995.

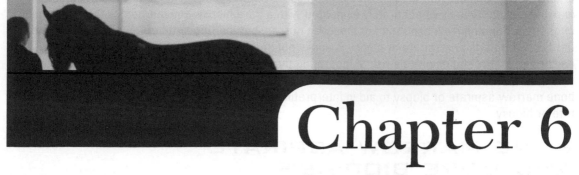

Chapter 6

BONE MARROW ASPIRATION AND CORE BIOPSY

Bone marrow of horses is easily aspirated or biopsied. An aspirate biopsy is easier to obtain than is a core biopsy. Cellular morphology is easier to assess on an aspirate smear, but evaluation of marrow cellularity is more accurately evaluated with a core biopsy. The sternum is the site usually chosen for bone marrow aspiration or biopsy in horses, but the ribs or tuber coxae are also potential sites. Although an aspirate or biopsy is easily obtained from the sternum, the procedure performed at this site involves a risk of lacerating the heart if the needle is inadvertently pushed through the sternebrae. Blood for a complete blood count should always be submitted along with a bone marrow aspirate or biopsy to aid in interpreting results of microscopic evaluation of the aspirate or biopsy.

BONE MARROW ASPIRATE AND CORE BIOPSIES

Indications

• To investigate abnormalities of the cellular components of blood, including unexplained anemia or polycythemia, thombocytopenia or thombocytosis, leukopenia or leukocytosis, or abnormal morphology of blood cells because reticulocytes are not released into peripheral circulation of horses, anemia can be classified as regenerative or nonregenerative only after cytologic examination of bone marrow.
• To determine body iron stores of anemic horses
• Bone marrow core biopsies are indicated when repeated attempts at aspiration are unsuccessful. Evaluation of a core biopsy may provide more accurate information than does an aspirate biopsy concerning cellularity of bone marrow.
• For collection of marrow for administration into a damaged tendon or ligament (i.e., autologous bone marrow therapy for tendinitis and desmitis)

Materials

• Several mL of local anesthetic solution (optional)
• The procedure can be performed more safely if sedation, local analgesia, or a lip twitch, or a combination of these aids is used.
• For a bone marrow aspirate biopsy, a biopsy/aspiration needle [e.g., a Jamshidi, Illinois Sternal, JorVet or Rosenthal bone marrow needle, 15- to18-ga (1.8- to1.2-mm)] (Figure 6.1) is used. An 18-ga, 3.5-in (1.2-mm, 8.89-cm), spinal needle is more often readily available and works well.
• For a bone marrow core biopsy, a larger biopsy/aspiration needle [8- to 11-ga (2.6 mm to 2.9 mm)] is used.
• Sterile surgical gloves, and a 12-mL or 20-mL syringe, with or without an anticoagulant (e.g., 10% EDTA or sodium citrate solution)
• Microscope slides
• 10% buffered formalin for a bone marrow core biopsy

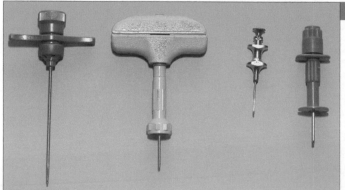

Figure 6.1

For aspiration of bone marrow, a 15- to 18-ga. needle is used. Shown in order from left to right are: Jamshidi, JorVet, Rosenthal, and Illinois Sternal needles. Biopsy of bone marrow is performed with a larger bore (8- to 11-ga.) needle.

BONE MARROW ASPIRATION

Procedure

• A local analgesic agent is injected subcutaneously at the *site of puncture, which is on the ventral midline, on or near a transverse line drawn between the points of the olecranons* (Figure 6.2). For tractable horses that are restrained with a lip twitch or sedation, the procedure can be performed safely without local anesthesia.

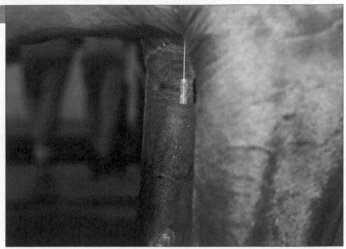

Figure 6.2

An 18-ga, 3.5-in (1.2-mm, 8.89-cm), spinal needle works well for aspiration of bone marrow. It is inserted into the sternum on a line connecting the points of the elbows.

• The bone marrow needle is inserted through skin and advanced until bone is encountered (Figure 6.3). The needle is pushed through the cortex of the sternebra by rotating the needle in an alternating clockwise and counter-clockwise motion. After the needle is advanced about 1-cm, the stylet is removed from the needle, the syringe is attached, and marrow is aspirated with a sharp pull on the plunger. If blood (i.e., marrow) is not obtained, the stylet is re-inserted, and the needle is rotated and pushed deeper.

• To avoid contaminating marrow with peripheral blood, only a few drops of marrow should be collected.

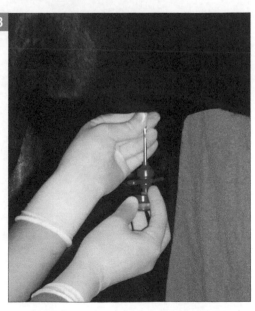

Figure 6.3

By rotating the needle in an alternating clockwise and counter-clockwise motion, the needle is pushed through the cortex of the sternebra.

- A drop of marrow is immediately (i.e., before it clots) placed on a microscope slide that is then tilted to allow contaminating blood to run off (Figure 6.4).
- A smear is made by placing a slide over the slide on which the aspirate was placed, the blood is allowed to spread, and the slides are pulled apart in a horizontal direction (Figure 6.5). The presence of particles on the microscope slides is evidence of a successfully performed bone marrow aspiration (Figure 6.6).
- Alternatively, marrow can be collected into a syringe containing 1 to 2 drops of EDTA anticoagulant for transport to a laboratory for processing. It is best to quickly process marrow collected in anticoagulant (i.e., within 1 hour), because the cells quickly deteriorate.
- Unfixed, air-dried slides can be submitted to the laboratory. Several slides should be submitted, because different stains may be used to evaluate the aspirate (e.g., Romanowsky stain for morphologic evaluation, Prussian blue stain for identification of iron stores).

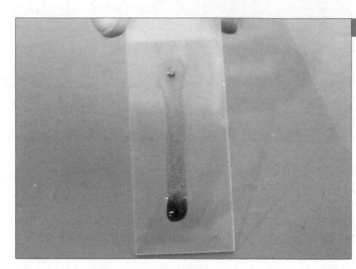

Figure 6.4

A drop of marrow is immediately (i.e., before it clots) placed on a microscope slide that is then tilted to allow contaminating blood to run off.

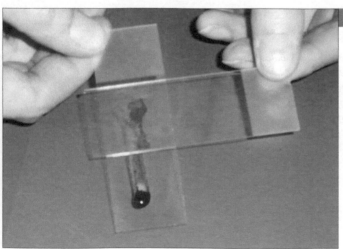

Figure 6.5

A smear is made by placing another slide over the slide on which the aspirate was placed, the sample is allowed to spread, and then the slides are pulled apart in a horizontal direction.

Figure 6.6

The presence of particles on the microscope slides is evidence of a successfully performed bone marrow aspiration.

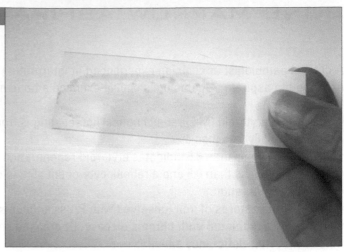

BONE MARROW CORE BIOPSY

Procedure

• The procedure is nearly the same as for aspiration, except that a larger needle [8-11-ga (2.6-mm to 2.9-mm) bone marrow biopsy/aspiration needle] is used, and the stylet is removed before the needle is advanced into bone.

• The biopsy needle is advanced until bone is encountered, the stylet is removed, and the biopsy needle is rotated as it is pushed approximately 1 cm deeper.

• The needle is then removed. The stylet is pushed through the needle tip, rather than the hub, to remove the tissue specimen from the needle (Figure 6.7).

• The specimen is placed in 10% neutral buffered formalin. (Before it is placed in formalin, it can be rolled across a glass side for cytological evaluation.)

Figure 6.7

For a bone marrow biopsy, the stylet is used to remove the tissue specimen from the needle by pushing the stylet through the needle tip rather than through the hub. The specimen is placed in 10% neutral buffered formalin.

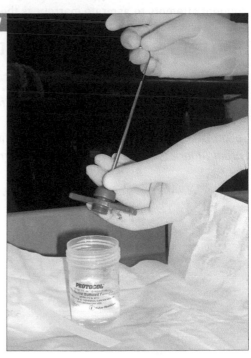

BONE MARROW ASPIRATE OR BIOPSY

Interpretation

A clinical pathologist or clinician experienced at interpreting bone marrow aspirates should examine the aspirate. A pathologist should examine a bone marrow biopsy.

• The myloid:erythroid (M:E) ratio of normal horses ranges from 0.5 to 1.5, and the marrow reticulocyte count is normally less than 5%.
• An M:E ratio less than 0.5 indicates erythroid regeneration or myloid suppression.
• An M:E ratio less than 0.5 and a reticulocyte count >5% is characteristic of a **regenerative anemia** of over 5 days duration.
• Bone marrow stores of iron (observed with Prussian blue stain) are normal or increased in horses with **anemia associated with chronic disease.** Decreased stores of iron are seen in marrow of horses with **iron-deficiency anemia.**
• Most leukemias originate in the bone marrow so any indication of leukemia on the CBC (unexplained increases or decreases or morphologic abnormalities in circulating leukocytes) can be confirmed by finding **neoplastic leukocytes** during examination of a bone marrow biopsy.
• Thrombocytopenia caused by increased consumption (disseminated intravascular coagulation or hemorrhage) or immune-mediated destruction is usually associated with normal to increased numbers or megakaryocytes in bone marrow. Decreased numbers of megakaryocytes are seen during examination of bone marrow of horses with **primary disease of bone marrow** (bone marrow aplasia or neoplasia).
• Replacement of bone marrow with fat that is observed during examination of biopsies taken from at least two sites substantiates a diagnosis of **bone marrow aplasia.**

Complications

• Complications are very rare, but *death from a needle-induced laceration of the heart can occur if the needle is accidentally pushed through the sternum.* This complication can be avoided by frequent attempts to aspirate marrow as the needle is advanced into the sternebra.

SUGGESTED READINGS

Henry MM. Diagnostic approach to anemia. In: Robinson NE, ed. *Current Therapy in Equine Medicine, 3rd ed,* WB Saunders Co, 1992, pp 487-492.

Sellon DC, Russell KE. The when, why and how of equine bone marrow analysis. *Proceedings 13th Forum American College of Veterinary Internal Medicine,* 1995, pp 604-607.

Harvey JW. *Atlas of Veterinary Hematology,* WB Saunders Co. Philadelphia, 2001, pp 96-123.

Chapter 7

COLLECTION OF
CORNEAL TISSUE

Corneal swabs and scrapings are collected from corneal ulcers for cytologic examination and bacterial or fungal culture and antimicrobial sensitivity testing. Corneal tissue should be examined cytologically when an immediate decision regarding therapy is needed, because cytological examination of corneal tissue often demonstrates the type of organism involved (e.g., gram-negative rods, gram-positive cocci or fungal hyphae). Culture medium inoculated with corneal tissue collected with a spatula often produces more bacterial growth than corneal tissue collected with a swab.

COLLECTION OF CORNEAL TISSUE

Indications
- For cytological analysis or bacteriological and fungal culture of a corneal ulcer that appears to be infected, has stromal melting, or is not responding to topical therapy. Clinical signs of infection include:
  - » corneal edema surrounding the ulcer
  - » miosis, epiphora, photophobia, and blepharospasm
  - » conjunctival and episcleral injection
  - » corneal neovascularization
  - » significant retention of rose bengal stain by the corneal epithelium in the absence of grossly visible corneal lesions or stromal uptake of fluorescein dye
  - » purulent ocular discharge
- When neoplastic disease (most commonly, squamous cell carcinoma) of the cornea is suspected.

Materials for Culture and Scraping
- Sedation and a lip twitch to prevent movement of the head
- Topical anesthetic solution, such as 0.5% proparacaine (Ophthaine, E.R. Squibb and Sons, Princeton, NJ; Alcaine, Alcon Laboratories, Fort Worth, TX) injectable anesthetic agents such as lidocaine HCL or mepivacaine HCL are not advised for topical anesthesia of the cornea, because these drugs are more toxic to corneal epithelium than are topical local anesthetic solutions intended for ophthalmic use. In addition, lidocaine and mepivacaine significantly inhibit bacterial growth, but proparacaine does not.
- Injectable local anesthetic solution (lidocaine HCL or mepivacaine HCL) for anesthesia of the auriculopalpebral nerve
- Sterile, rayon- or cotton-tipped swabs synthetic-tipped swabs are preferred because cotton-tipped swabs contain fatty acids that inhibit bacterial growth.
- Transport medium (e.g. Amies or Stuart's medium), or thioglycollate broth and Sabouraud dextrose agar for direct culture
- Sterile spatula (Kimura Spatula, Storz Instruments) and an alcohol-type burner for resterilization between multiple scrapings, or a sterile scalpel blade
- Glass microscope slides
- Cold packs for transport

Procedure
- The horse should be adequately sedated and a lip twitch applied to minimize the danger of additional corneal damage during the procedure.
- An auriculopalpebral or palpebral nerve block facilitates the procedure. The auriculopalpebral nerve can be anesthetized with 5mL of local anesthetic solution administered at a depth of 2 cm in a depression palpated at a junction where the dorsal border of the zygomatic process of the temporal bone meets a line drawn along the posterior border of the ramus of the mandible. Or alternatively, one to 2mL of local anesthetic solution is injected subcutaneously over the palpebral branch of the nerve where it can be palpated as it crosses the dorsal aspect of the zygomatic arch halfway between the lateral canthus of the eye and the base of the ear (Figure 7.1).

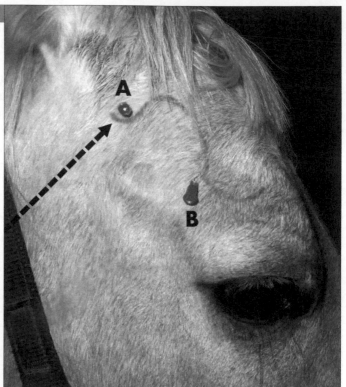

Figure 7.1

An auriculopalpebral nerve block facilitates the corneal scraping. The nerve can be anesthetized by administering local anesthetic solution in a depression palpated where the dorsal border of the zygomatic process of the temporal bone meets a line drawn along the posterior border of the ramus of the mandible. (A). Or alternatively, local anesthetic solution is injected subcutaneously over the palpebral branch of the nerve where it can be palpated as it crosses the dorsal aspect of the zygomatic arch halfway between the lateral canthus of the eye and the base of the ear (B).

• Several drops of a topical anesthetic solution are sprayed on the cornea using a syringe attached to the hub of a small gauge needle that has had its shaft removed (Figure 7.2). Some ophthalmologists advise that corneal swabs and scrapings intended for microbiological culture be performed *without* topical anesthesia of the cornea because topical anesthetic solutions interfere with bacterial survival. It may be difficult, however, to collect a corneal swab or scraping from a horse without corneal anesthesia, and proparacaine has minimal deleterious effect on growth of pathogenic bacteria.

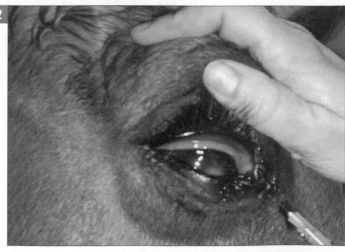

Figure 7.2

Several drops of a topical anesthetic solution are sprayed on the cornea using a syringe attached to the hub of a small gauge needle with the shaft removed.

• If a culturette swab (Culturette, Marion Scientific, Kansas City, MO) is used, the swab should be moistened with the swab's transport medium *before* the swab's package is opened. The likelihood of culturing an organism is increased if a moist swab is used. Breaking the ampule of transport medium moistens the swab.

• The swab is applied to the edge of the corneal lesion and then inoculated onto thioglycollate broth and Sabouraud dextrose agar for direct microbiological culture, or the swab is placed in a transport medium (e.g., Amies or Stuart's medium) and placed on a cold pack for transport.

• Edges of the corneal lesion are scraped with a spatula or the blunt end of a scalpel blade (Figures 7.3 & 7.4), and the tissue obtained is spread on a glass slide and air-dried. If possible, multiple smears should be prepared. A drop of a 10 to 20% solution of potassium hydroxide (KOH) applied to a fresh smear (i.e., before it dries) facilitates identification of fungi. A minimum staining routine should include Gram's and Giemsa stains.

• Tissue from the corneal scraping is also placed in transport medium (e.g. Amies or Stuart's medium) or inoculated into thioglycollate medium and Sabouraud dextrose agar for direct culture.

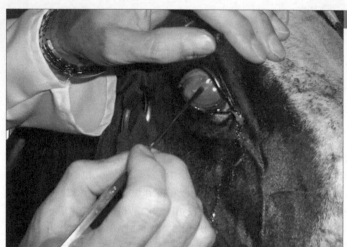

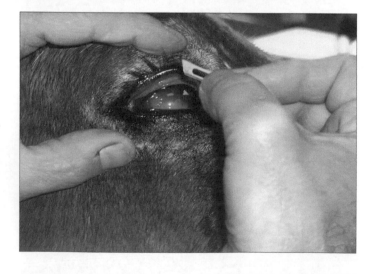

Figures 7.3 & 7.4

Edges of the corneal lesion are scraped with a spatula or the blunt end of a scalpel blade.

CYTOLOGICAL OR MICROBIOLOGIC FINDINGS

Interpretation

- Gram-negative rods seen during cytological examination indicates the possibility of infection with *Pseudomonas* sp.
- Most fungi are detectable by Gram's staining.
- A diagnosis of keratomycosis cannot be ruled out by negative cytological or microbiologic findings.

SUGGESTED READINGS

Slatter D. *Fundamentals of Veterinary Ophthalmology* WB Saunders Co., Philadelphia, 2001, pp101-103.

Brooks DE. *Ophthalmology for the Equine Practitioner* (Made Easy Series), Teton NewMedia, Jackson WY, 2002.

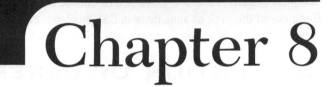

Chapter 8

COLLECTION OF CEREBROSPINAL FLUID (CSF)

Analysis of CSF seldom supplies an etiologic diagnosis of neurologic disease. In some instances, analysis of cerebrospinal fluid may provide clues that when combined with history, physical examination, and other diagnostic procedures, may aid in diagnosis or management of horses with neurologic disease. Cerebrospinal fluid should be collected from the site closest to the lesion, if possible, at either the atlanto-occipital cistern or the lumbo-sacral cistern. The lumbo-sacral cistern is the site preferred to collect CSF in horses with signs of spinal cord disease, and the atlanto-occipital cistern is the site preferred to collect CSF from horses with signs of brain disease. Because of the lack of sensitivity in CSF analysis, collecting CSF from the appropriate site may improve the chances that analysis will provide useful information.

COLLECTION OF CEREBROSPINAL FLUID (CSF)

Indications
• Collection of CSF is indicated for horses with neurologic disease, when information gained from CSF analysis could potentially influence case management.

Contraindications
• CSF should not be collected from horses suspected of having rabies.
• Collection of CSF is contraindicated for horses with head trauma or metabolic disease that have signs of significant cerebral edema (such as dilated pupils and an altered state of consciousness). Removal of CSF from a horse with elevated intracranial pressure may cause a rapid decrease in CSF pressure resulting in death from herniation of brain tissue through the *foramen magnum*. This complication is rare.
• Collection of CSF from the atlanto-occipital cistern requires general anesthesia and therefore contraindicated for horses that are at risk of dying under general anesthesia, or of being unable to regain a standing position.
• Puncture of the *dura mater* by the spinal needle is painful and may provoke an extreme reaction in the standing horse, which could cause injury to the clinician or horse. Collection of CSF from the lumbo-sacral cistern is contraindicated if the temperament of the horse or an inadequate facility to restrain the horse jeopardizes the safety of the clinician or horse.

Materials
• To collect CSF from the atlanto-occipital cistern of an adult horse, an 18- to 20-ga (1.2- to 0.9-mm), 3.5-in (8.89-cm) needle with a stylet is used. For foals, a 20-ga 1.5-in (3.8 cm) disposable hypodermic needle without a stylet can be used to collect CSF from the atlanto-occipital cistern. To collect CSF from the lumbo-sacral cistern of an adult horse, an 18-ga (1.2-mm), 6 to 8-in (15.24- to 20.32-cm) needle with a stylet is used. (A 6-in. needle is sufficiently long for a 450-500 kg horse with normal body condition.) For foals, an 18- to 20-ga, 3.5-in. (8.89-cm) needle with a stylet is used at the lumbo-sacral site.
• Sterile gloves
• 10 mL syringe
• #11 blade or 16-ga needle (optional)
• General anesthesia is required to collect fluid from the atlanto-occipital cistern, and local anesthetic solution is used to collect fluid from the lumbo-sacral cistern.
• Sedation may dampen the reaction to puncture of the *dura mater* at the lumbo-sacral site in the standing horse, but sedation may compound the difficulty of persuading an already ataxic horse to stand squarely to facilitate accurate placement of the needle. To dampen the reaction to puncture of the *dura mater,* a lip twitch should be applied to a standing horse, even if the horse is sedated.

• EDTA tubes. Microproteins can now be accurately measured in CSF collected into EDTA tubes. Because the low protein concentration of CSF causes cellular destruction, CSF collected in plain glass tubes should be examined within 30 minutes.
• Enrichment media for bacterial culture, if indicated
• Cold packs for shipment of samples. CSF should be kept cold for shipment. Cytology of CSF collected in EDTA tubes should be performed within 24 hours.

COLLECTION AT THE LUMBO-SACRAL SITE

Procedure

• The site for needle placement is identified on the midline between the cranial borders of the *tuber sacrale.* This landmark is difficult to identify in a well-conditioned horse, and the approximate site can be identified on a line drawn between the caudal borders of the *tuber coxae* on the midline (Figure 8.1).
• The site is surgically prepared, and local anesthetic solution is injected subcutaneously.
• The horse should be persuaded to stand squarely, if possible.

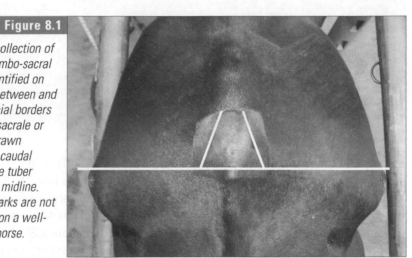

Figure 8.1

The site for collection of CSF at the lumbo-sacral cistern is identified on the midline between and near the cranial borders of the tuber sacrale or near a line drawn between the caudal borders of the tuber coxae on the midline. These landmarks are not easily found on a well-conditioned horse.

• Puncturing the skin with a #11 blade or a large bore needle reduces drag on the spinal needle as it is advanced.
• The spinal needle is advanced in a vertical plane when viewed from the side and from behind. The needle is usually advanced at least 5in (11.2cm) before the *dura mater* is penetrated. Entry into the lumbo-sacral cistern usually elicits **a reaction from the horse that can be violent,** especially if the needle is rapidly advanced. If the needle is advanced slowly, a milder reaction (e.g., tail flagging, and arching of the back) is more likely.
• The stylet is removed from the needle, and fluid is gently aspirated from the subarachnoid space. Excessive suction may result in blood contamination of the sample.
• If there is no reaction during advancement to bone, and fluid can not be aspirated, the stylet should be reinserted and the needle pulled to a subcutaneous position for reinsertion, or completely removed for reinsertion at a location 1.5cm caudad or craniad from the original point of insertion.
• Ensuring that the hind limbs are parallel and pulled forward facilitates collection of CSF from the lumbo-sacral cistern of a laterally recumbent horse. Pulling the hind limbs forward enlarges the lumbo-sacral space.

COLLECTION AT THE ATLANTO-OCCIPITAL SITE

Procedure

• The horse is anesthetized, placed in lateral recumbency, and the area for needle placement is prepared for aseptic insertion of the needle.

• The neck is positioned parallel with the ground surface, and the head is flexed so that the median axis of the head is at a right angle to the cervical vertebrae.

• The site for needle placement for collection of CSF is at the atlanto-occipital cistern on the dorsal midline of the neck, on an imaginary transverse line drawn between cranial borders of the wings of the atlas (Figure 8.2).

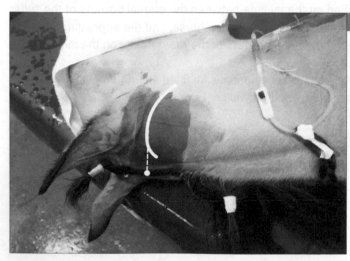

Figure 8.2

The site for needle placement for collection of CSF at the atlanto-occipital cisternis on the dorsal midline of the neck, on an imaginary transverse line drawn between cranial borders of the wings of the atlas (white line).

• A styleted needle is inserted perpendicular to the skin surface and parallel with the ground surface and advanced as if aiming for the commissure of the lips. The bevel of the needle should be directed rostrally. For foals, a hypodermic needle without a stylet can be used.

• Penetration into the subarachnoid space can be appreciated as a popping sensation and loss of resistance at 5 to 8 cm in adult horses and at 2 to 4 cm in foals. CSF should be observed to flow from the needle after the stylet is removed; if not, the stylet is replaced, and the needle is advanced further. CSF is collected by allowing it to flow into a collection tube (Figure 8.3).

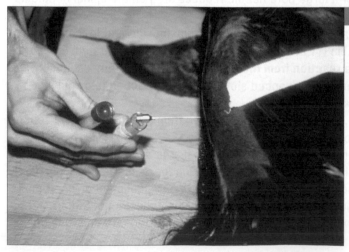

Figure 8.3

CSF is collected from the atlanto-occipital cistern by allowing it to flow into a collection tube.

CSF

Interpretation

• CSF is normally **clear and colorless. Opacity** indicates either a high cell count or an abnormally high protein concentration. High protein concentration may cause CSF to have a **foamy appearance.**
• Normal **protein concentration** ranges from 20 to 80 mg/dL in adults and up to 180 mg/dL in foals.
• CSF normally has a **cell count** of less than 8 mononuclear cells /uL. Red blood cells are not normally present. Increased numbers of mononuclear cells are typical of viral disease of the CNS, and a neutrophilic pleocytosis is typical of bacterial or parasitic disease of the CNS. Eosinophils, which are not present in CSF from normal horses, may be seen with parasitic disease of the CNS.
• **Red-tinged** CSF indicates either traumatic injury to the CNS or blood contamination from trauma during the tap (Figure 8.4). CSF that has become contaminated with blood during the tap often clears as the fluid continues to flow from the needle, but CSF remains red-tinged if blood in the CSF was caused by CNS injury. The *presence of platelets* in the sample of CSF indicates iatrogenic RBC contamination. Absence of red cells does not rule out trauma as a cause of neurological signs.
• **Yellow-tinged** CSF (xanthochromia) results from the presence of blood pigments and indicates prior hemorrhage or leakage of blood from inflamed blood vessels. Xanthochromic CSF is a typical finding in horses with equine herpesvirus myeloencephalitis. CSF of extremely icteric horses may also be xanthochromic. CSF of normal neonates may be slightly xanthochromic.

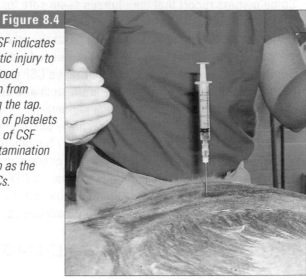

Figure 8.4

Red-tinged CSF indicates either traumatic injury to the CNS or blood contamination from trauma during the tap. The presence of platelets in the sample of CSF indicates contamination during the tap as the source of RBCs.

• **Black-tinged** CSF indicates the presence of a melanoma within the CSF.
• CSF collected for **detection of antibodies to *Sarcocystis neurona* for diagnosis of equine proto-zoal myelitis** has limited value. CSF that is **negative** on immunoblot assay for antibodies to *Sarcocystis neurona* is a good indication that neurologic disease is not associated with infection of this organism, but CSF of some affected horses, in the early stages of disease, may be negative on immunoblot assay. CSF that is **positive** on immunoblot assay for antibodies to *Sarcocystis neurona* is not diagnostic for *S. neurona* for several reasons:

» Because most horses, in endemic areas, have been exposed to *S. neurona* and have serum antibodies for this organism, blood-contaminated CSF of these horses may be positive for *S. neurona* antibodies. Contamination of CSF with blood during collection is possible, and probably common, even without gross evidence of contamination. Commonly used methods for determining if CSF is blood-contaminated (i.e., the albumin quotient, the IgG index, and the red blood cell count) may not identify a blood-contaminated sample.

» Any neurologic disease that causes a break in the blood-brain barrier of a horse that has anti-*S. neurona* serum antibodies, might allow passage of those antibodies into the CSF.

» *S. neurona* organisms might be present in the CNS in insufficient numbers to cause clinical signs yet may evoke an antibody response (i.e., subclinical infection).

» Antibodies might persist in the CSF long after the horse has recovered from clinical or subclinical infection.

• CSF collected for **detection of *Sarcocystis neurona* DNA (i.e., polymerase chain reaction testing) for diagnosis of equine protozoal myelitis** has limited value, because the test is usually negative in horses affected with equine protozoal myelitis. The parasite is an intracellular organism and is unlikely to be found in CSF.

• Activity of CSF **creatine phosphokinase,** an enzyme found in myelin, is not helpful in evaluation of horses with neurologic disease, because contamination of CSF with epidural fat and dura can contribute to increased activity of this enzyme.

Complications

• Needle placement may be attempted numerous times before the subarachnoid space at the lumbosacral site is penetrated. An owner who observes the procedure should be warned of this possibility and assured that complications from numerous attempts are unlikely.

• A violent reaction by the horse to penetration of the *dura mater* at the lumbo-sacral site may result in injury to the horse or people involved in the procedure.

• Some owners report that their horses seem sore for several days after CSF is collected at the lumbo-sacral site.

• General anesthesia for collection of CSF at the atlanto-occipital site carries its own risks, and horses with neurological disease have increased risk of injury during recovery from anesthesia.

• Removal of CSF from horses with increased CSF pressure caused by cerebral edema may relieve pressure, resulting in damage to the brain stem and death caused by herniation of the cerebrum and cerebellum through the *foramen magnum.*

• Contamination of CSF with blood is a likely occurrence during collection of CSF. Iatrogenic hemorrhage (gross or microscopic) in the CSF may be difficult to differentiate from hemorrhage associated with disease. Blood-tinged CSF containing iatrogenic hemorrhage is likely to have a heterogeneous distribution and tends to clear as CSF is withdrawn. When hemorrhage is associated with disease, CSF is likely to be xanthochromic after centrifugation.

• Failure to use aseptic technique during collection of CSF may result in septic meningitis.

SUGGESTED READINGS

Miller MM, Sweeney CR, Russell GE, Sheetz, RM, Morrow JK. Effects of iatrogenic blood-contaminated equine CSF on *Sarcocystis neurona* western blot reactivity and CSF indices. *Proceedings, 44th Annual Convention American Association Equine Practitioners* 44:138-139, 1998.

Bernard WV. Equine protozoal myelitis - laboratory tests and interpretation. *International Equine Neurology Conference,* College of Veterinary Medicine, Cornell University, July 11-13, 1997, pp 7-9.

Johnson PG, Constantinescu GM. Collection of cerebrospinal fluid in horses. *Equine Vet Edu* 2:13-20, 2000.

Johnson PG, Constantinescu GM. Analysis of cerebrospinal fluid in horses. *Equine Vet Edu* 2:21-26, 2000.

MacWilliams PS. Cerebrospinal fluid. In: Cowell RL, Tyler RD., eds. *Cytology and Hematology of the Horse.* Goleta, CA. American Veterinary Publications: 1992:171:179.

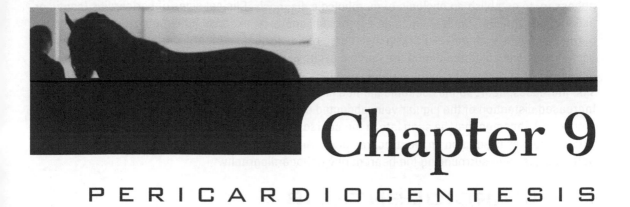

Chapter 9

PERICARDIOCENTESIS

Pericardial disease in the horse is rare, but when it is suspected, collecting pericardial fluid may be necessary to establish an etiologic or morphologic diagnosis. Clinical signs of pericarditis (septic or aseptic) are variable, but often include depression, anorexia, exercise intolerance, dyspnea, tachycardia, tachypnea, and fever. Early in the course of the disease, pericardial friction rubs can sometimes be auscultated during the cardiac cycle; pericardial friction rubs indicate that a small amount of fluid is in contact with a roughened pericardial surface. As the volume of pericardial effusion increases, heart sounds become muffled and friction rubs, if previously present, may disappear. Increased distention of the jugular vein, abducted elbows, and edema of the ventral portion of the thorax and abdomen may be seen late in the course of the disease. Decreased amplitude of the QRS complexes is seen on an electrocardiogram. Anechoic or hyperechoic fluid, often containing fibrin tags, is seen surrounding the heart during echocardiography.

PERICARDIOCENTESIS

Indications
• For cytologic evaluation, to determine if fluid has accumulated because of bacterial infection, trauma, neoplasia, or is idiopathic
• For bacterial culture and antimicrobial sensitivity testing (although pericardial fluid should be cultured for both aerobic and anaerobic bacteria, isolating a causative agent is unlikely)
• To remove pericardial effusion, which may also produce immediate clinical improvement
• To insert a catheter for repeated pericardial drainage and lavage
• To infuse antimicrobial drugs into the pericardial space

Contraindications
• Septic pleuritis (may introduce infection into pericardial space)
• External wounds overlying the site of centesis. (The procedure can usually be performed from either side of the thorax.)

Materials
• Sedation (may be contraindicated when the horse has signs of cardiac tamponade, such as tachypnea and tachycardia)
• #15 blade and sterile gloves
• 2 to 3mL mepivacaine HCl
• A 12- to 14-ga (2.64- to 2.03-mm), intravenous catheter or teat cannula. A 12- to 32-french thoracic tube can be inserted and secured *in situ* if the pericardial sac is to be repeatedly drained or lavaged.
• 60-mL syringe
• Bacterial transport medium
• EDTA and plain glass collection tubes
• Ultrasonographic equipment for selection of the optimal site for pericardiocentesis (strongly advised)
• Electrocardiographic monitoring equipment to detect arrhythmias that may develop during the procedure
• Fluids for intravenous administration during drainage of the pericardial sac, if the horse has signs of cardiac tamponade, such as tachycardia or tachypnea
• Warm, sterile, balanced electrolyte solution or physiological saline solution for lavage of the pericardial sac

Procedure

- Usually performed with the horse standing
- Preferably, the **horse is electrocardiographically monitored** during the procedure.
- May be performed on either side, **preferably with ultrasonographic guidance,** but the left side is most frequently used. The choice of right side or left side depends on the likelihood of puncturing the lung during pericardiocentesis, as determined by ultrasonography.
- Pericardiocentesis is usually performed at **the left 5th or 6th intercostal space,** in an area above the olecranon and below a horizontal line through the point of the shoulder (Figure 9.1).

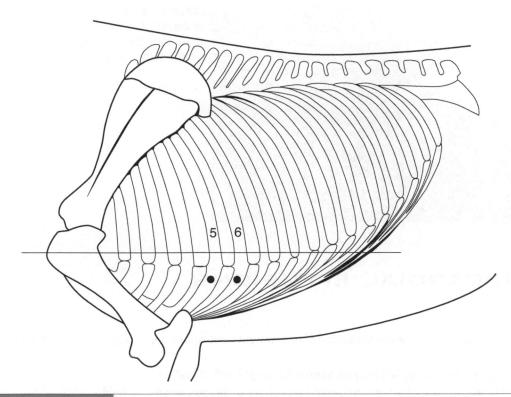

Figure 9.1 *Pericardiocentesis is usually performed at the left 5th or 6th intercostal space, in an area above the point of the elbow and below a horizontal line through the point of the shoulder.*

- After surgical preparation of the skin, local anesthetic solution is injected subcutaneously and into the intercostal muscle at the proposed site of aspiration.
- A 0.5-cm cutaneous incision is made using a #15 blade. The incision may be longer, if a thoracic tube is being inserted for pericardial drainage. The incision should be made at the cranial edge of a rib to avoid the intercostal vessels.
- The catheter or cannula, with the syringe attached, is advanced into the thorax in **a horizontal plane and aimed cranially at a 30° angle.** During advancement, gentle negative pressure is applied to the syringe. When the heart, or thickened pericardium is touched, movement of the heart can usually be appreciated. Fluid should flow into the syringe as soon as the pericardial sac is penetrated. Aspiration of fluid may not be possible if the pericardium is adhered to the heart.

• The pericardial sac should be drained slowly, especially if the horse has signs of cardiac tamponade (Figure 9.2).
• Pericardial lavage can also be performed at this time. If sepsis is suspected, an antimicrobial drug (avoid the use of procaine penicillin G or a highly ionic drug) can be instilled into the pericardial sac before the catheter is removed.
• The skin incision can be left to heal as an open wound.

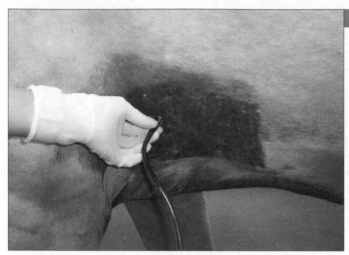

Figure 9.2

The pericardial sac should be drained slowly, especially if the horse has signs of cardiac tamponade.

PERICARDIAL EFFUSIONS

Interpretation

• Indications of sepsis are the presence of degenerate neutrophils and a protein concentration >2.5 g/dL.
• Nondegenerate neutrophils may be seen with aseptic inflammation.
• Microorganisms are often not recovered on culture of septic pericardial fluid.
• Neoplastic cells may occasionally be observed in pericardial effusion obtained from horses with neoplasia of the pericardium.
• Eosinophils are seen in pericardial fluid of horses with a type of idiopathic pericarditis that responds favorably to treatment with corticosteroids.

Complications

• Irritation/laceration of the myocardium or left descending coronary artery (causing arrhythmia or hemorrhage, either of which may result in death)
• Catheter/needle breakage
• Contamination of the pleural cavity with septic pericardial fluid or neoplastic cells.

SUGGESTED READING

Reef VB. Cardiovascular system examination. In: Orsini JA and Divers TJ, eds., *Manuel of Equine Emergencies, Treatment and Procedures.* WB Saunders Co., Philadelphia, 1998, pp 94-156.

Chapter 10

SINOCENTESIS

Sinocentesis is performed to collect fluid from the paranasal sinuses for diagnostic purposes and to create a portal for lavage. The most common clinical signs of disease of the paranasal sinuses are unilateral nasal discharge, epiphora, decreased airflow and malodor from the nares of the affected side, a dull sound during sinus percussion, and facial swelling of the affected side of the head. *Fluid for cytological examination is most commonly aspirated from the caudal maxillary sinus,* because this is the paranasal sinus most likely to contain fluid when there is disease of the paranasal sinuses. The contents of the caudal maxillary sinus can be sampled directly with a catheter or by inserting a catheter through the frontal sinus and fronto-maxillary aperture into the caudal maxillary sinus. The ventral conchal sinus and rostral maxillary sinus do not communicate directly with the caudal maxillary sinus, and consequently the rostral maxillary sinus must be sampled when disease of the rostral maxillary or ventral conchal sinuses is suspected.

SINOCENTESIS

Indications
- When clinical signs and endoscopic or radiographic findings indicate disease of the paranasal sinuses.
- To collect fluid for gross visual examination for detection of a sinus cyst
- To collect fluid for cytological examination, bacterial culture, and antimicrobial sensitivity
- To introduce fluid for lavage of the paranasal sinuses
- For biopsy of masses identified during radiographic examination
- For sinoscopy, which involves insertion of an arthroscope or endoscope into the paranasal sinuses

Contraindications
- There are few, if any, contraindications for sinocentesis.

Materials
- #15 scalpel blade and sterile gloves
- Sedation is optional
- 2 to 3mL mepivacaine HCl
- Battery-operated drill and bit; or a Steinmann pin and hand chuck; or a 16-ga (1.6-mm), steel needle and hammer
- Catheter (such as a dog urinary catheter or a male cat urinary catheter) and syringe for aspiration of fluid
- Sterile, physiologic saline solution
- An alligator-type ronguer, if a biopsy is to be performed.
- Bacterial transport medium for culture of exudate or 10% formalin for a biopsy sample, as indicated
- Microscope slides for cytological examination of fluid

Procedure
- Performed with the horse standing
- The site of sinocentesis is chosen (Figure 10.1). The location of the maxillary septum, which separates the rostral and caudal maxillary sinuses, varies but it usually lies directly over the second molar. For most horses, the septum is 2/3 of the distance from the medial canthus of the eye to the rostral aspect of the facial crest. The variable location of the septum (Figure 10.2) can cause confusion as to which sinus has been sampled during sinocentesis. But because all compartments communicate directly or indirectly, the site of sampling may be inconsequential.

1) In general, *direct* centesis of the **caudal maxillary sinus** can be performed at a site 2 cm rostral and 2-3 cm ventral from the medial canthus of the eye. *Indirect* centesis of the caudal maxillary sinus can be performed over the frontomaxillary aperture in the conchofrontal sinus at a site half to 2/3 of the distance from the facial midline to the medial canthus of the eye.

2) Because the **rostral maxillary sinus** varies in size and location, centesis of this sinus should be performed only after radiographic determination of its location and only if there is radiographic evidence of disease in the rostral or ventral conchal sinus *(the rostral maxillary sinus and the ventral conchal sinus communicate through the conchomaxillary aperture).* Centesis of the rostral maxillary sinus often can be performed at a site 60% of the distance (along the facial crest) from the medial canthus of the eye to the rostral aspect of the facial crest and 1cm ventral to a line from the infraorbital foramen to the medial canthus of the eye. The *levator nasolabialis* muscle should be reflected dorsally prior to drilling through the *maxillary* bone.

Figure 10.1

*Sites for sinocentesis are depicted in this drawing. **A** = direct centesis of the caudal maxillary sinus; **B**= indirect sinocentesis of the caudal maxillary sinus; **C**= sinocentesis of the rostral maxillary sinus (location of this site may vary and is best determined with a radiograph).*

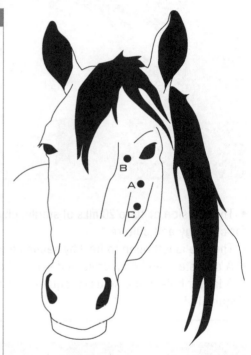

Figure 10.2

The location of the maxillary septum (arrow), which separates the rostral and caudal maxillary sinuses, varies. The variable location of the septum can cause confusion as to which sinus has been sampled during sinocentesis.

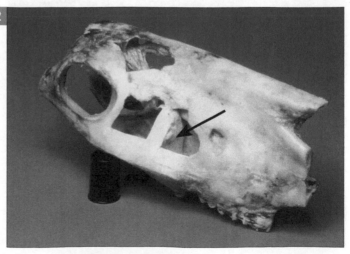

• After surgical preparation of the proposed site of sinocentesis, the skin and subcutaneous tissue is infiltrated with a local anesthetic solution (facial bone has little sensation).

• The skin, subcutaneous tissue, and periosteum are incised in a longitudinal plane with a #15 scalpel blade. A hole in the bone, large enough to accommodate the catheter, is made using a sterile drill bit, Steinmann pin, or a 14- (2.03-mm) or 16-ga (1.6-mm), steel needle (Figure 10.3). For the rostral maxillary sinus, in particular, the pin should protrude no more than 0.5 cm from the hand-chuck to avoid damage to apices of the cheek teeth or infraorbital canal.

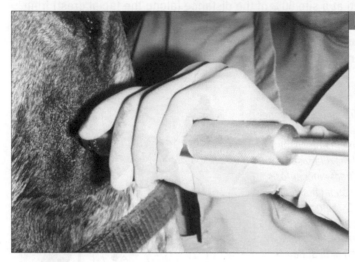

Figure 10.3

A hole in the bone, large enough to accommodate a dog urinary catheter or a male cat urinary catheter, is made using a sterile drill bit, Steinmann pin, or a 16-ga (1.6-mm), steel needle.

• The infusion of 10 to 20 mLs of sterile, physiologic saline solution may facilitate aspiration of fluid for cytology and culture.

• The site is left open to heal by second intention or closed with staples or a suture.

• A catheter can be inserted and secured for daily lavage, if necessary (Figure 10.4).

• A larger hole in the sinus is required for insertion of a Foley catheter, arthroscope, or endoscope (Figure 10.5).

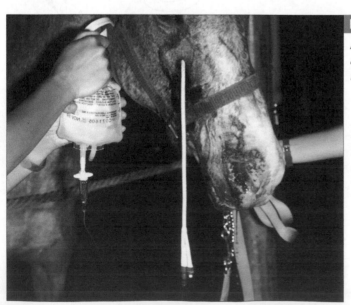

Figure 10.4

A catheter can be inserted and secured for daily lavage, if necessary.

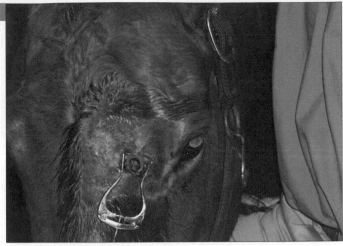

Figure 10.5

A larger hole in the sinus is required if insertion of a Foley catheter, arthroscope, or endoscope is indicated.

SINUS ASPIRATE

Interpretation

- In cases of **secondary sinusitis,** many different species of bacteria may be found during cytological examination or from culture of aspirated fluid. Plant material may sometimes be found during cytological examination, when sinusitis is caused by dental disease. Fluid is usually malodorous when sinusitis is caused by dental disease or neoplasia.
- In cases of **primary sinusitis,** either no bacteria or only a single species of bacteria, usually a streptococcal species, is found during cytological examination or from culture of aspirated fluid. Fluid may be malodorous, especially if the sinuses contain inspissated exudate.
- A viscid, amber fluid is characteristic of a **sinus cyst** (Figure 10.6).

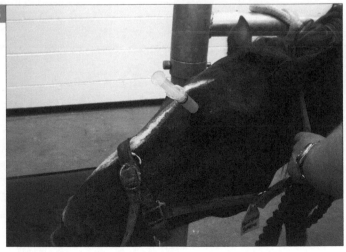

Figure 10.6

A viscid, amber fluid is characteristic of a sinus cyst.

Complications

- Serious complications are rare.
- Cellulitis may occur at the site of centesis, in which case, the horse may require antimicrobial therapy.
- Subcutaneous emphysema is usually localized and resolves spontaneously.

• Damage to the apices of the cheek teeth, resulting in periapical infection. This complication is most likely to occur in young horses during centesis of the rostral maxillary sinus.

• Epistaxis may occur if highly vascular structures, such as the ethmoid labyrinth are perforated inadvertently. Hemorrhage may appear to be severe, but usually resolves spontaneously.

SUGGESTED READINGS

Laverty S, Pascoe JR. Sinusitis. In: Robinson, NE. ed: *Current Therapy in Equine Medicine 4,* WB Saunders, 1997, pp 419-421.

Nickels FA. Nasal passages. In: Auer JA, Stick JA. eds: *Equine Surgery, 2nd ed.* WB Saunders, 1999, pp. 326-336.

Trumaine WH, Dixon PM. A long-term study of 227 cases of equine sinonasal disease. Part 1: Details of horses, historical, clinical and ancillary diagnostic findings. *Equine Veterinary Journal* 33:274-282, 2001.

Trumaine WH, Dixon PM. A long-term study of 227 cases of equine sinonasal disease. Part 2: Treatments and results of treatments. *Equine Veterinary Journal* 33:283-289, 2001.

Chapter 11

THORACOCENTESIS

Horses with signs of pleural disease should undergo thoracocentesis to obtain pleural fluid for cytological and bacteriological analysis. Clinical signs of pleural disease include signs of pain such as pawing, reluctance to move, stiff gait, and abducted elbows and, rarely, subcutaneous edema of the pectoral and sternal regions. Affected horses may have evidence of pleural effusion, such as absence of lung sounds in the ventral portion of the thorax, tachypnea, dyspnea, and a change in resonance during thoracic percussion. As the volume of pleural effusion increases, heart sounds may radiate into the dorsal thoracic region. Thoracic ultrasonographic examination or thoracocentesis verifies the presence of thoracic effusion. Radiographic examination should not be necessary for diagnosis of pleural effusion, but rather should be used as an aid to determine the cause of thoracic disease **after** drainage of the thorax.

THORACOCENTESIS

Indications
- To verify the presence of pleural effusion suspected during clinical examination
- To collect fluid for cytological evaluation to determine if the fluid has accumulated because of infection, inflammation, trauma, or neoplasia
- To collect fluid for bacterial culture and antimicrobial sensitivity testing
- To remove pleural effusion, blood, or air responsible for respiratory distress.
- For local therapy

Contraindications
- External wounds over the site of thoracocentesis

Materials
- Sedation facilitates the procedure
- #15 blade and sterile surgical gloves
- 5 to10mL of mepivacaine HCl
- 14 ga intravenous catheter **or**
- Teat cannula, bitch urinary catheter **or**
- An indwelling chest tube, if repeated or continuous drainage is indicated. For continuous drainage, a Heimlich valve (Becton Dickinson, Lincoln Park, NJ) or finger from exam glove or condom, with the tip removed (to attach to the chest tube to prevent aspiration of air) is also needed.
- 10 to 20 mL syringe to attach to the catheter or teat cannula **or**
- Stopcock for attachment to the cannula or catheter
- Intravenous extension set (optional, but may be attached to teat cannula to guide drainage into a bucket)
- Transport medium for aerobic and anaerobic bacterial culture of pleural fluid
- EDTA and plain glass collection tubes to collect fluid for cytological examination
- Ultrasonography can be used to locate the optimal site for fluid collection and drainage and to reduce the risk of contact between the heart and cannula or catheter. Such contact can induce fatal cardiac arrhythmia.

Procedure
- Performed with the horse standing
- Sedation is usually not necessary and, for some horses, may be contraindicated.
- Descriptions of the site for thoracocentesis vary, but these descriptions identify similar sites: **The 6th, 7th or 8th intercostal space,** just above the palpable bulge of the costochondral junction and dorsal to the lateral thoracic vein (on a horizontal line drawn from point of the shoulder), is usually chosen for thoracocentesis (Figure 11.1).

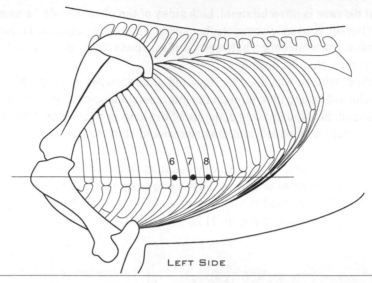

LEFT SIDE

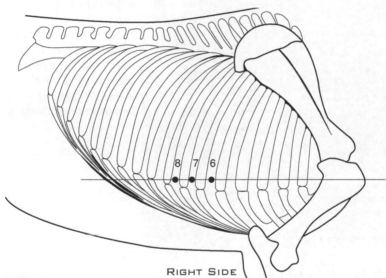

RIGHT SIDE

Figure 11.1   *Descriptions of the site for thoracocentesis vary, but these descriptions identify similar sites. For either side, the 7th or 8th intercostal space is most commonly entered.*

• After scrubbing the skin, local anesthetic solution is infiltrated subcutaneously and deep into the intercostal muscle.

• A 0.5cm skin incision is made through the skin parallel to the ribs using the #15 blade. A slightly longer incision is made if a chest tube is to be inserted for thoracic drainage. The incision should be made at the cranial edge of a rib to avoid the intercostal vessels and nerves.

• A blunt teat cannula, to which a syringe or stopcock has been attached, to prevent the introduction of air into the thorax, or a chest tube is carefully inserted into the chest cavity. A "popping" sensation is usually noted as the cannula or chest tube penetrates the pleura. Entry can be ascertained by periodically applying negative pressure until fluid is obtained. Subcutaneous tunneling of the cannula or chest tube has been recommended to minimize aspiration of air, but this technique may cause a chest tube to kink and increases the difficulty of the procedure.

• The fluid sample is collected in the syringe and transferred to the collection tubes and transport medium.

• **Because pleural disease is often bilateral, both sides of the chest should be sampled.** The mediastinum of mature horses is usually complete, but immature horses have small mediastinal perforations that allow communication between cavities. These perforations may plug with fibrin and cellular debris when pleuritis develops.

• An **indwelling chest tube** may be used for repeated or continuous drainage. More force is required to punch the indwelling tube through the intercostal muscles than is required with the teat cannula. Caution should be used to avoid puncture of the lung or heart. When the tube is in the thoracic cavity, the trocar is removed, and drainage should start immediately. The chest tube should be attached to the skin with sutures, such as the Chinese lock stitch, to prevent accidental removal. Pleural fluid should be allowed to drain passively because suction often results in obstruction of the drainage portals. A Heimlich valve or a finger from a latex glove, or a condom from which the tip has been removed should be applied to the chest drain to create a one-way valve, which allows drainage but prevents pneumothorax (Figure 11.2).

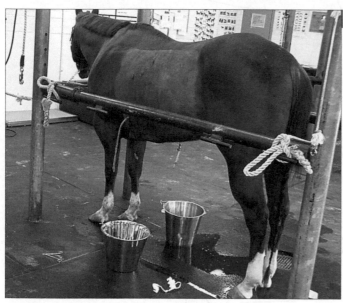

Figure 11.2

A Heimlich valve, or a finger from a latex glove, or a condom from which the tip has been removed should be applied to the chest drain to create a one-way valve, which allows drainage but prevents pneumothorax.

PLEURAL FLUID

Interpretation

• Normal pleural fluid is straw-colored, clear, and odorless. Normally, no fluid or only a small volume (<10ml) is collected, but up to 100mL can be collected from normal horses.

• Protein concentration is normally less than 3 gm/dL.

• Cell count is normally less than 10,000 cells/uL, most of which are non-degenerate neutrophils; the remainder is mononuclear and mesothelial cells.

• Indications that pleural fluid is septic are:
   » a cell count >10,000 cells /uL (the cell count may be within normal range, despite sepsis),
   » the presence of degenerate neutrophils,
   » a cloudy fluid that often contains fibrin clots,
   » a foul odor (this indicates anaerobic infection and a poor prognosis for survival),
   » a protein concentration greater than 3gm/dL (although concentrations greater than this have been reported in normal horses),
   » a glucose concentration <40mg/dL.

• A preponderance of morphologically normal lymphocytes indicates a chylous effusion, whereas a preponderance of morphologically abnormal lymphocytes is an indication of lymphosarcoma.

Complications

- Cellulitis at the site of centesis
- Penetration of the abdominal cavity and enterocentesis can occur when thorococentesis is attempted at the most caudal recommended sites, especially when the cannula or catheter is directed caudoventrally.
- Pneumothorax. This complication can be prevented by careful placement of the cannula or chest tube and proper use of a one-way valve.
- Puncture of lung or heart. The thorax should be ultrasonographically or radiologically examined to determine the position of the heart, which may have shifted, because of large volumes of fluid or thoracic masses.

SUGGESTED READINGS

Schott HC, Mansmann RA. Thoracic drainage in horses. *Compendium of Continuing Education for the Practicing Veterinarian.* 12: 251-261, 1990.

Beech J. Thoracocentesis, pleuroscopic examination, and lung biopsy. In: Beech, J. ed. *Equine Respiratory Disorders.* Lea and Febiger, Philadelphia, pp.63-68, 1991.

Chapter 12

COLLECTION OF LOWER AIRWAY SECRETIONS

Secretions from the lower airways can be collected for cytological evaluation and culture by several methods. Tracheal aspirates (also called tracheobronchial aspirates) can be collected through tubing placed into the trachea percutaneously (transtracheally) [i.e., a **transtracheal aspiration (TTA)**] or through the accessory channel of an endoscope. Secretions from the lower airways also can be collected by aspiration of fluid infused directly into a bronchus [i.e., a **bronchoalveolar lavage (BAL)**]. Cytological evaluation of fluid collected by BAL is superior to cytological evaluation of fluid collected by TA for diagnosis of diffuse pulmonary disease, but fluid collected by BAL is less suitable for bacterial culture.

TRANSTRACHAEL ASPIRATION

• Because the nasopharynx of normal horses harbors pathogenic and nonpathogenic bacteria and fungi, airway secretions collected by an endoscope introduced into the trachea through the nasal passage and nasopharynx is more likely to be contaminated with *microorganisms* than is a sample obtained by TTA. A TTA also is less likely to be contaminated with *cells* from the nasopharynx, which, especially in the case of upper airway inflammation, could confuse the cytologic interpretation.

Indications
• For collecting secretions from the lower portion of the respiratory tract, when identification of infectious microorganisms is particularly important.

Materials
• A lip twitch (optional for some horses)
• Sedation with xylazine or butorphanol may facilitate the procedure by dulling the cough reflex.
• A commercial needle, and catheter kit (Jorgensen Laboratories, Inc.1450 N. Van Buren Ave., Loveland Co. 80538), **or** a homemade kit using a large-bore hypodermic needle with appropriately sized polyethylene (PE) tubing (Intramedic Polyethylene Tubing, Clay Adams, Becton Dickinson & Co, Parsippany NJ 07054)
    » #190 PE tubing fits through a 13-ga needle; an 18-ga needle (Monoject Blunt Cannulas, Tyco Healthcare Group LP. Mansfield, MA) fits into this tubing.
    » #205 PE tubing fits through a 12-ga needle. A16-ga needle fits into this tubing.
    » a stiff PE tube such as a French #5 dog urinary catheter (Tyco Healthcare Group LP. Mansfield, MA) fits through the lumen of a 12-ga hypodermic needle and is easier to manipulate and is less likely to be severed by the needle than is soft PE tubing (Figure 12.1).

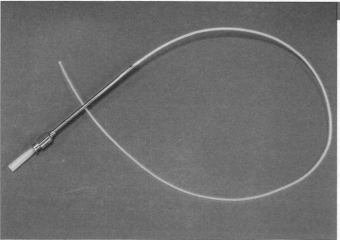

Figure 12.1

For performing a TTA, a stiff PE tube such as a No. 5 dog urinary catheter fits through the lumen of a 12-ga hypodermic needle and is easier to manipulate and is less likely to be severed by the needle than is soft PE tubing.

- Sterile, physiological saline solution and a 20-to 60-mL syringe
- #15 scalpel blade (optional)
- Materials to prepare a sterile site
- One mL of local anesthetic solution
- An EDTA tube for submission of a sample for cytological examination or glass slides for immediate preparation of an obviously highly cellular aspirate
- Transport media suitable for both aerobic and anaerobic culture.

Procedure

- Skin at the junction of the lower one-third and upper two-thirds of the neck over the trachea is scrubbed, and local anesthetic solution is injected subcutaneously at the proposed site of puncture.
- A longitudinal stab incision is made on the midline between tracheal rings, if the rings can be palpated.
- The needle is inserted horizontally into the trachea between rings with the bevel pointed down, while stabilizing the trachea with one hand (Figure 12.2). As soon as the needle tip enters the trachea, the hub is lifted and the needle is advanced down the trachea. Ability to easily aspirate air with a syringe indicates correct placement of the needle. Care should be taken to avoid lacerating the opposite wall of the trachea with the needle.

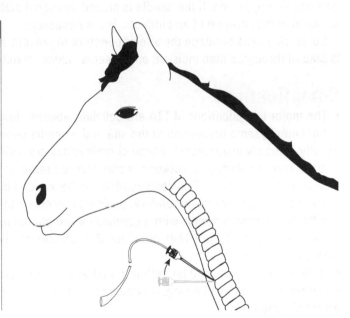

Figure 12.2

For a TTA the needle is inserted horizontally into the trachea between rings with the bevel pointed down. As soon as the needle tip enters the trachea the hub is lifted and the needle is advanced.

- The catheter is advanced through the needle to, or past the horizontal portion of the trachea at the thoracic inlet. At this stage of the procedure, some clinicians prefer to remove the needle from the horse to prevent the possibility of accidentally severing the PE tubing. By leaving the needle in place for the entire procedure, however, the likelihood of contaminating the subcutaneous tissue with pathogenic bacteria is lessened.
- Twenty to 60mL (20mL for foals) of sterile physiological saline solution is injected through a blunt hypodermic needle that fits tightly in the catheter (by an ungloved assistant) (Figure 12.3). Aspiration should be started immediately after injection is complete. If an aspirate is not obtained, more saline solution is injected for aspiration. Often, only a small amount of the saline solution can be retrieved.
- After aspiration the catheter is pulled gently back through the needle. If the needle tip catches the catheter, the needle and catheter are retracted together to avoid severing the catheter.

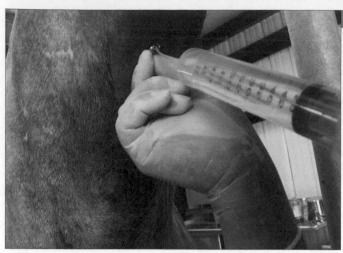

Figure 12.3

For adult horses 60mLs of saline is infused through the catheter. If an insufficient quantity of saline for cytology and culture is aspirated, aliquots of 60 mL of saline are infused until sufficient quantity is aspirated.

• Some clinicians inject an antibiotic, such as gentamicin or penicillin, subcutaneously at the site of needle puncture to avoid cellulitis that could occur from contamination of subcutaneous tissue with pathogenic organisms. If the needle is placed through a stab incision, cellulitis seldom results, and so, local administration of an antibiotic is not necessary.
• Some clinicians bandage the site of puncture to prevent subcutaneous emphysema. If the needle is placed through a stab incision, emphysema seldom results, and so, a bandage is not necessary.

Complications

• The major complications of TTA are cellulitis, abscess formation, and subcutaneous and mediastinal emphysema originating at the site of the needle puncture. The latter two complications are usually clinically insignificant. *These complications are unlikely to occur if the needle is advanced into the trachea through a cutaneous stab incision rather than through a puncture.*
• Severing the catheter. This complication can be avoided by keeping the bevel of the needle pointed downward for the procedure, pulling the needle if the catheter catches on the point of the needle, or by using a needle with a cannula for the procedure. A severed catheter is usually coughed out within minutes (Figure 12.4), but if not, the catheter can be retrieved using an endoscope and its biopsy instrument.
• If the catheter is passed up, rather than down the trachea, it may enter the oral cavity where it can be damaged by chewing. A chewed catheter can be very difficult to retrieve through the tracheal puncture.

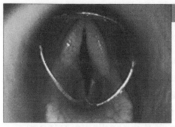

Figure 12.4

A severed catheter is usually coughed out within minutes, but if not, the catheter can be retrieved using an endoscope and its biopsy instrument.

TRACHEAL ASPIRATION THROUGH AN ENDOSCOPE

• A disadvantage of this method of tracheal aspiration is that the endoscope may carry secretions of the upper airway into the trachea, causing erroneous interpretation of microbiological and cytological findings. The accessory port of the endoscope may harbor bacteria that interfere with interpretation of microbiological findings. A tracheal aspirate obtained using an endoscope is less likely to be contaminated if a commercially available guarded aspiration catheter is utilized.

Indications

• When culture of microorganisms from secretions from the lower respiratory tract is less important than cytological evaluation of the secretions
• When a skin wound or the risk of complications that can develop from the transtracheal method of obtaining the aspirate are unacceptable to the owner of the horse

Materials

• An **unguarded** endoscopic flushing catheter (Endoscopic Flushing Catheter, SurgiVet, Waukesha, WI) or 180 to 240cm of PE tubing that fits easily through the accessory channel of an endoscope (PE 240 tubing for an 11-mm endoscope or PE 190 tubing for a 9-mm endoscope.) **Or:** A commercially available, **guarded**, endoscopic tracheal catheter may decrease the likelihood of contamination with upper airway secretions (Endoscopic Microbiology Aspiration Catheter, Mila International, Inc., 510 West South St., Covington, KY 41011) (Figure 12.5).

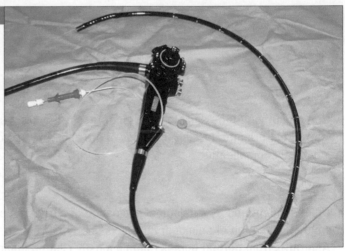

Figure 12.5

For tracheal aspiration using an endoscope, a commercially available, guarded, endoscopic tracheal catheter may decrease the likelihood of contamination with upper airway secretions.

• A hypodermic needle that tightly fits the PE tubing for injection of sterile, physiologic saline solution. Sterile, blunt needles that are less likely to cut the PE tubing are commercially available (Monoject Blunt Needles, Sherwood Medical, St. Louis MO 63103) or can be made by blunting a hypodermic needle.
• Sterile, physiological saline solution and a 20- to 60-mL syringe
• EDTA collection tubes for submission of the aspirate for cytological evaluation or microscope slides for immediate preparation of an obviously cellular aspirate
• Transport media suitable for aerobic and anaerobic bacterial culture. *An aspirate obtained using an endoscope is unsuitable for culture unless a guarded catheter is used to obtain the sample.*
• Sedation or a lip twitch may be necessary to restrain some horses, especially young horses. Sedation with xylazine, detomidine or butorphanol may also facilitate the procedure by dulling the cough reflex.

Procedure

• The PE tubing is passed through the accessory channel of the endoscope until the tube appears at its end. The insertion tube of the endoscope containing the PE tubing is passed through a nasal passage to the cranial thoracic region of the trachea where there is a dependent area in which respiratory secretions collect.

• The PE tubing (or the inner catheter of a guarded catheter) is advanced into any visible pool of exudate, which is then aspirated (Figure 12.6).

• Or sterile, physiological saline solution is infused through the tubing and then aspirated by maneuvering the tubing into pools of saline solution.

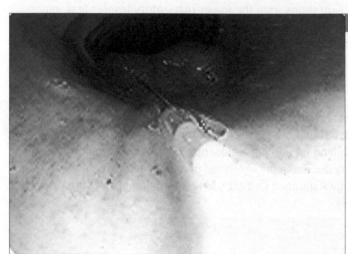

Figure 12.6

During a tracheal aspiration using an endoscope, sterile, physiological saline solution is infused through polyethylene tubing and then aspirated by maneuvering the tubing into pools of saline solution.

Complications

• Contamination of the sample with upper respiratory tract secretions invalidates the results of bacterial culture and possibly, cytology of the aspirate. Use of guarded catheters lessens the likely-hood of this complication.

Interpretation

• Disease identified by cytological evaluation of a tracheal aspirate and disease identified by histological examination of pulmonary tissue is poorly correlated.

• Aspirates from **normal horses** contain mostly ciliated columnar epithelial cells, mononuclear cells, and few neutrophils [stabled horses normally have more neutrophils (e.g., 20% neutrophils) than do pastured horses (e.g., 5% neutrophils)].

• Finding of stratified squamous epithelial cells indicates contamination of the aspirate with secretions from the upper regions of the respiratory tract (Figure 12.7). The presence of these cells invalidates results of bacterial culture. Depending on the severity of contamination, cytology of the aspirate may be difficult to interpret.

• Fungal elements can be found in the aspirates of normal horses.

• Aspirates of **horses with bacterial bronchopneumonia** contain predominately neutrophils that are often degenerate (Figure 12.8). A large number of *intracellular* bacteria is highly suggestive of a septic process. If processing of the sample is delayed, however, extracellular bacteria become phagocytized and multiply in respiratory secretory cells.

Figure 12.7

Finding of squamous epithelial cells (arrows) invalidates bacteriological results of a tracheal aspirate because presence of these cells indicates contamination of the aspirate with secretions from the upper regions of the respiratory tract. Bacteria (probably a contaminate from the pharynx) can be seen on one of the epithelial cells.

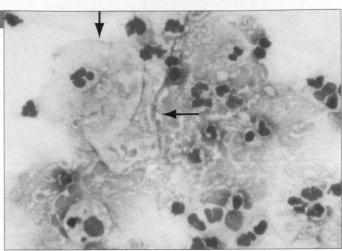

Figure 12.8

Tracheal aspirates of horses with bacterial bronchopneumonia contain predominately neutrophils that are often degenerate.

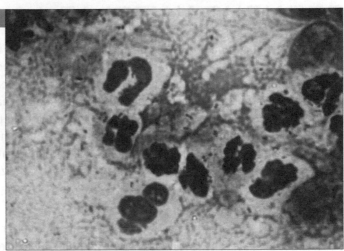

• Aspirates of **horses with recurrent airway obstruction (heaves)** contain large numbers of morphologically normal neutrophils, and mucus is plentiful. Curschmann's spirals (inspissated mucus with a coiled appearance) are occasionally seen (Figure 12.9).

• Aspirates of **horses with recent exercise-induced pulmonary hemorrhage** contain RBCs. For several weeks after an occurrence of exercise-induced pulmonary hemorrhage, macrophages with intracytoplasmic hemosiderin can be found in aspirates.

• Unless a guarded catheter was used to obtain the sample, bacteria cultured from an aspirate obtained with an endoscope are likely to be contaminates.

• Because bacteria can be cultured from transtracheal aspirates of normal horses, culturing of bacteria from a tracheal aspirate is significant only if,

    a) cytological findings support a diagnosis of sepsis (e.g., inflammatory exudate composed of degenerate neutrophils that contain intracellular bacteria).

    b) clinical findings support a diagnosis of sepsis (e.g. fever, anorexia, depression, abnormal sounds heard during thoracic auscultation, etc.)

    c) cultured bacteria are established respiratory pathogens.

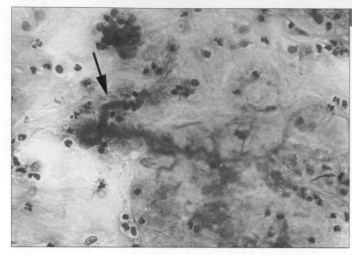

Figure 12.9
Tracheal aspirates of horses with heaves contain large numbers of morphologically normal neutrophils and plentiful mucus. Curschmann's spirals (inspissated mucus with a coiled appearance) are occasionally seen (arrow).

BRONCHOALVEOLAR LAVAGE

• Bronchoalveolar lavage (BAL) is easily performed and the BAL fluid (BALF) retrieved provides information concerning cell populations in peripheral air spaces that correlates well with cell populations found in lung tissue obtained by biopsy or during necropsy. Because BAL samples secretions from only a small segment of lung, focal lung disease may not be recognized using this procedure. When focal lung disease (e.g., exercise-induced pulmonary hemorrhage, pneumonia, lung abscess, or neoplasia) is suspected, fluid retrieved from a TA is more likely to aid in diagnosis. BAL can be performed using an endoscope or a catheter that is passed blindly. Using an endoscope for BAL is advantageous, because endoscopy allows visualization of the bronchus to be sampled.

Indications
• For cytological examination of secretions of small peripheral airways and alveolar spaces, especially when lung disease is mild or only suspected, and is likely to be diffuse

Materials
• A 180-cm (or longer) endoscope for horses and a 150-cm endoscope for ponies. The diameter of the endoscope determines the size or generation of bronchus sampled. Or a commercially available, catheter designed for the purpose of BAL (Broncho-alveolar lavage catheter, Bivona Co., Gary, IN; Broncho-alveolar lavage catheter, Cook Veterinary Product, Inc., 501 N Rogers Street, Bloomington, IN).
• Profound sedation (using xylazine or detomidine combined with butorphanol) is advised to inhibit the cough reflex or, alternatively, less sedation combined with use of a diluted local anesthetic solution (injection of 25 to 30mLs of lidocaine diluted with an equal amount of saline) instilled though the accessory channel or catheter as the scope or catheter is passed.
• Lip twitch
• A 10-mL syringe is used to inflate the cuff of a lavage catheter.
• 5, 60-mL syringes filled with sterile, warm or room temperature, physiological saline solution; if saline is warmed to body temperature, less bronchospasm results during infusion and thus more saline is retrieved.

- A method of processing aspirated fluid:
  a) Cytocentrifigation is the usual method of processing BALF, but because cytocentrifuges are expensive, **BALF samples are best submitted to a laboratory for cytocentrifigation.**
  b) Or a basic laboratory centrifuge is used to concentrate cells so that slides can be made.
  c) Or **40% or 50% ethanol** (or another fixative recommended by the laboratory) is added to the BALF to fix cells.

Procedure

- BAL is most easily performed when the horse is **heavily sedated** and restrained with a lip twitch, but for some horses the procedure can be performed without sedation.
- The endoscope or catheter is passed through a nasal passage and down the trachea until it becomes wedged in a bronchus. Holding the horse's **head in extension** facilitates blind passage of the catheter through the nasopharynx into the trachea. Using an oral speculum may prevent damage to the catheter if the catheter is inadvertently passed to the mouth rather than the trachea (Figure 12.10).

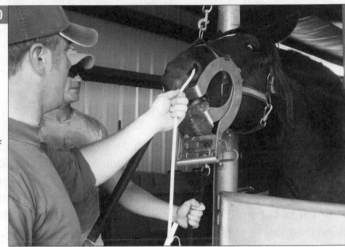

Figure 12.10

Holding the horse's head in extension facilitates blind passage of the catheter through the nasopharynx into the trachea. Using an oral speculum may prevent damage to the catheter if the catheter is inadvertently passed to the mouth rather than the trachea.

- Three hundred mLs of warm or room temperature, physiological saline solution is infused through the accessory channel of the endoscope or the catheter and then aspirated with 60-mL syringes. (Alternatively, infusion of as little as 80mLs physiological saline solution is claimed to be sufficient for BAL.) **Recovery of 50% to 90% of the lavage solution is expected.** Recovery of less than 40% of the lavage fluid indicates that the catheter or endoscope failed to completely occlude the bronchus [i.e., insufficient cuff inflation or failure to prevent the endoscope or catheter from shifting from its wedged position (e.g., during coughing)]. Small amounts of fluid may be retrieved from horses with severe heaves because these horses often develop bronchospasm during the procedure. The surface layer of aspirated fluid should have a **foamy appearance,** because of its surfactant content, if the BAL catheter was placed properly (Figure 12.11). A layer of foam may not be present if the catheter was improperly placed or for some horses with severe recurrent airway obstruction.
- Aliquots of aspirated lavage solution are mixed and submitted to a laboratory for processing for cytological examination. Or:
  a) If BAL samples cannot be processed within 3-4 hours, the fluid should be refrigerated or chilled on ice. Chilled or refrigerated BALF should be processed within 24 hours.
  b) BAL samples can be centrifuged (1500 rpm for 5 min) and a smear made from the cell pellet that remains after the supernatant is decanted. These dried smears can be submitted to the laboratory.

c) BAL fluid can be mixed with an equal volume of 40% or 50% ethanol (100-proof vodka is 50% ethanol) or another fixative recommended by the laboratory. *Special stains are required* for cytological evaluation of cells from fluid mixed with ethanol and *morphology of cells fixed with ethanol is difficult to interpret.*

• BAL fluid usually is not submitted for bacteriological examination because the catheter or endoscope becomes contaminated with microorganisms from the nasopharynx during its passage to the lower airways.

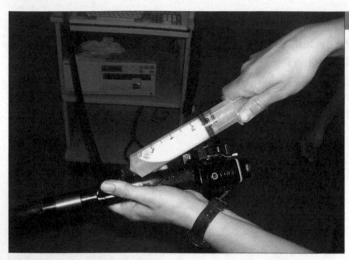

Figure 12.11

The surface layer of aspirated fluid should have a foamy appearance, because of its surfactant content, if the BAL catheter was properly placed.

Interpretation

• Normal BALF is clear or slightly turbid with a foamy layer of surfactant on its surface. A layer of foam may not be present if the catheter was improperly placed or for some horses with severe recurrent airway obstruction. Flocculant material indicates the presence of mucus and cellular debris. A reddish or brownish color of BALF indicates recent or old pulmonary hemorrhage, respectively.

• Because various descriptions of BAL recommend using different volumes of fluid for infusion, published values of total nucleated cell counts and differential counts of cells contained in BAL samples vary slightly. When 100 to 300 mLs of fluid is used for lavage, cytological results are similar.

• In a recent study, there was no significant difference in total nucleated or differential cell counts of sequential or pooled aliquots of BALF. Therefore, each aliquot of BALF can be considered to represent the cytology of the lavaged lung segment, and recovery of even a small amount of fluid is likely to be of diagnostic value.

• **Macrophages** and **lymphocytes** are the most common cells found in BAL samples retrieved from normal horses.

• A concentration of more than 5% **neutrophils** is found in BAL samples of horses with heaves, viral respiratory disease, or bacterial pneumonia (in horses with bacterial pneumonia, the neutrophils are degenerate) or lower airway inflammation of young racehorses. More neutrophils are seen in BALF when a small volume of saline is used.

• A concentration of more than 5% **eosinophils** is found in BAL samples retrieved from horses with respiratory parasitism, idiopathic, eosinophilic, immune-mediated pulmonary diseases, young racehorses with lower airway inflammation, and rarely, horses with recurrent airway obstruction (Figure 12.12).

• Viral infections are the usual cause of increased numbers of **ciliated epithelial cells in BALF** that normally account for less than 5% of the cell population.

• **Hemosiderophages** are normally found in BAL samples of horses that exercise strenuously.

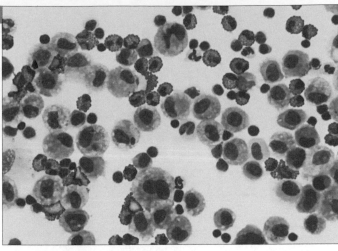

Figure 12.12

A concentration of more than 5% eosinophils is found in BAL samples retrieved from horses with respiratory parasitism, idiopathic eosinophilic immune-mediated diseases, and rarely, horses with heaves.

• BALF of young racehorses with lower airway inflammation (a.k.a. small airway disease or inflammatory airway disease) often contains increased numbers of either **mast cells** (i.e., > 4%) or eosinophils or both, or neutrophils.

Complications
• Complications are rare, but include mild coughing, depression, and fever. Some clinicians suggest that strenuous exercise should be avoided for several days after the procedure.

SUGGESTED READINGS

Beech J. Tracheobronchial aspirates. In: Beech J. (ed.) *Equine Respiratory Disorders.* Lea and Febiger, Philadelphia, pp.41-53, 1991.

McGorum BC, Dixon, PM. The analysis and interpretation of equine bronchoalveolar lavage fluid (BALF) cytology. *Equine Veterinary Education* 6:203-209, 1994.

Mansmann RA, King C. How to perform bronchoalveolar lavage in practice. *Proceedings, 44th Annual Convention American Association Equine Practitioners* 44:186-188, 1998.

Hinchcliff KW, Byrne BA. Clinical examination of the respiratory system. *Veterinary Clinics of North America: Equine Practice* 7:1-26, 1991.

Hoffman AM. Bronchoalveolar lavage technique and cytological diagnosis of small airway inflammatory disease. *Equine Veterinary Education* 1:208-214, 1999.

Mair T. Diagnostic techniques for lower respiratory tract diseases. In: Robinson NE. (ed.) *Current Therapy in Equine Medicine 3rd Ed.* WB Saunders Co., Philadelphia pp.299-303, 1992.

Pickles K, Pirie RS, Rhind S, Dixon PM, McGorum BC. Cytological analysis of equine bronchoalveolar lavage fluid. Part 1: comparison of sequential and pooled aliquots. *Equine Veterinary Journal* 34:288-291, 2002.

Pickles K, Pirie RS, Rhind S, Dixon PM, McGorum BC. Cytological analysis of equine bronchoalveolar lavage fluid. Part 2: comparison of smear and cytocentrifuged preparations. *Equine Veterinary Journal* 34:292-296, 2002.

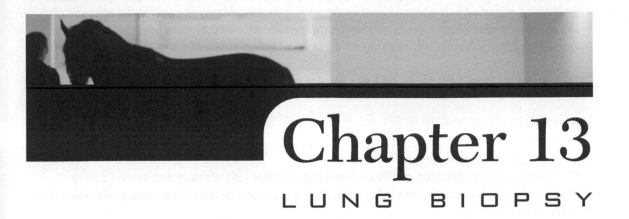

Chapter 13

LUNG BIOPSY

Lung tissue can be obtained by **transthoracic biopsy** or by **transbronchial biopsy.** These procedures are seldom performed in the horse because transthoracic lung biopsy is considered by many clinicians to be a dangerous procedure and histology of tissue obtained by transbronchial biopsy is poorly described for horses with pulmonary disease.

TRANSTHORACIC LUNG BIOPSY

Indications
• For histological identification of focal pulmonary masses discovered during thoracic radiographic or ultrasonographic examination
• For histological identification of diffuse, interstitial nodular lung disease discovered during thoracic radiographic examination (e.g., for definitive diagnosis of interstitial pneumonia when this disease is suspected)
• When material for fungal or bacterial culture is required
• When less invasive methods have failed to supply a diagnosis, if diagnosis is essential to determine the treatment and prognosis of a horse affected with pulmonary disease

Contraindications
• Rapid and irregular, or labored respiration or violent and uncontrollable coughing increase the risk of lacerating the lung with the biopsy needle
Some clinicians consider the following diseases also to be contraindications of transthoracic lung biopsy:
• Pulmonary abscesses, pneumonia, and pleuropneumonia
• Exercise-induced pulmonary hemorrhage
• Recurrent airway obstruction (heaves)

Materials
• #15 blade and sterile gloves
• 3 to 5mL of local anesthetic solution
• A manually operated, Tru-Cut style biopsy needle can be used, but use of an automated, spring-loaded biopsy device (Bard Monopty Biopsy Instrument, Bard Peripheral Technologies, 1383 Harland Drive N. E., Covington GA. 30014) may increase the safety of the procedure.
• Ultrasonographic equipment for selection of biopsy site (optional)
• Microscope slides, 10% formalin and media for transport of tissue for fungal and bacterial culture if needed

Procedure
• Sedation is optional, but restraint should be such to prevent movement during the procedure.
• When radiographic or ultrasonographic evaluation is not used to determine the optimal site for biopsy, a site commonly used is the 7th or 8th right intercostal space, approximately 8 cm above a horizontal line through the olecranon. The 7th or 8th intercostal space on or above a horizontal line drawn through the scapulohumoral joint is another site recommended for lung biopsy. Lung biopsy can be performed from either side of the chest, but the risk of cardiac or great vessel rupture is claimed to be less if the biopsy is taken from the right side.
• Other intercostal spaces are also used for lung biopsy. The risk of lacerating blood vessels of significant size may decrease if the biopsy is taken superficially and from the caudodorsal lung field (Figure13.1).

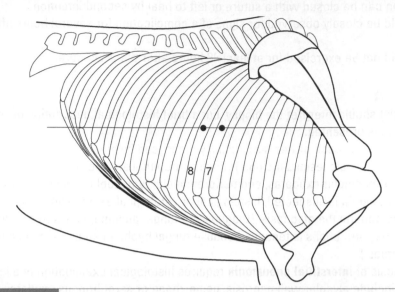

Figure 13.1 *When radiographic or ultrasonographic evaluations are not used to determine the optimal site for biopsy, a site commonly used is the 7th or 8th right intercostal space, approximately 8 cm above a horizontal line through the humeroradial joint.*

- After preparing the biopsy site for aseptic insertion of the biopsy needle, the body wall, down to and including parietal pleura, is infiltrated with local anesthetic solution, and the skin is stabbed with a #15 blade near the cranial edge of the neighboring rib. (That site avoids the intercostal vessels located at the caudal edge of each rib.)
- The biopsy needle is placed into the incision and then advanced a small distance through the chest wall and into lung parenchyma. Because of the elastic nature of lung, the specimen notch of the needle often only partially fills with lung tissue (Figure 13.2). More lung tissue may be obtained by using a spring-loaded, automated biopsy needle rather than a manually operated Tru-Cut style needle. *To minimize trauma to the lung that can occur with chest movement, the sample should be taken immediately after insertion of the needle into lung.* Several samples of lung should be obtained.
- An impression smear can be made from a sample before it is placed in formalin. Another sample can be placed in a bacterial transport medium.

Figure 13.2

Because of the elastic nature of lung, the specimen notch of the needle only partially fills with lung tissue. More lung tissue may be obtained by using a Biopty® needle rather than a manually operated Tru-Cut style needle.

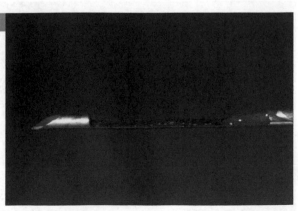

- The stab incision can be closed with a suture or left to heal by second intention.
- The horse should be closely observed for signs of a complication for several hours after the procedure.
- The horse should not be exercised for at least 48 hours after the procedure.

Interpretation

- A histopathologist should interpret the biopsy, but a brief histological description of some pulmonary diseases is presented.
- **Recurrent airway obstruction or heaves** is usually diagnosed by means other than lung biopsy, but expected histopathologic lesions include bronchiolar epithelial hyperplasia, goblet cell hyperplasia/metaplasia, bronchiolar exudates, and peribronchiolar lymphoplasmacytic infiltration.
- When **fungal pneumonia** is suspected, histological or cytological examination, or culture of a lung biopsy sample may confirm the diagnosis. (Diagnosis of fungal pneumonia based on cytological examination of airway secretions is tenuous because fungal hyphae can be found in airway secretions of normal horses.)
- Definitive diagnosis of **interstitial pneumonia** requires histological examination of a lung biopsy. Expected lesions include alveolar wall necrosis, hemorrhage or serofibrinous exudates within alveoli, desquamation of pneumocytes, and interstitial inflammation and fibrosis. In some affected foals, a necrotizing bronchiolitis is also seen (**bronchointerstitial pneumonia**).
- A granulomatous, interstitial pneumonia and, in some cases, small, refractile, crystalline particles within macrophages may be seen during histological examination of lung of horses with **silicate pneumoconiosis.**
- Pulmonary **neoplasia** is usually localized, and negative biopsy findings do not rule out this disease.

Complications

The incidence of death of horses after transthoracic lung biopsy was 3% in one survey. Because complications of transthoracic lung biopsy are common and occasionally fatal, this procedure should be performed only after other less hazardous techniques have failed to supply information essential for a diagnosis that may influence treatment. Owners should be informed of potential complications associated with transthoracic lung biopsy.

Reported complications are:

- **Clinical signs of pulmonary hemorrhage** (coughing, hemoptysis, epistaxis, tachycardia, collapse, and, occasionally, death) (Figure 13.3). The incidence of this complication is estimated to be 6 to 10%.

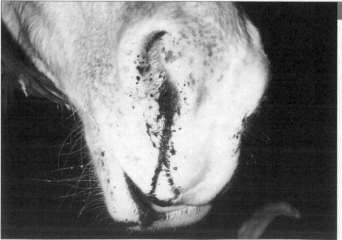

Figure 13.3

Coughing with hemoptysis, epistaxis, tachycardia, collapse, and death is an occasional complication of lung biopsy in the horse.

- **Pneumothorax** (clinical signs are tachypnea and dyspnea). This complication is uncommon, and affected horses rarely require treatment.
- **Neurogenic shock** (sudden collapse). Most horses recover rapidly from this complication.
- **Fatal air embolism** associated with lung biopsy is reported to occur in people and is a potential complication for horses undergoing lung biopsy.
- **Failure to obtain diseased tissue.** Unless lung disease is diffuse or can be biopsied using ultrasonic guidance, obtaining tissue of interest is unlikely.

TRANSBRONCHIAL LUNG BIOPSY

Although the procedure for transbronchial lung biopsy has been described, we are unaware of any studies that correlate histological findings or culture results with findings using other techniques of diagnosis of pulmonary disease.

Materials
- An 180cm long (or longer) endoscope for horses and a 150cm long endoscope for ponies
- An endoscopic biopsy forceps. By using a biopsy forceps that has a spike between the biopsy cups to prevent the jaws of the forceps from sliding, full-thickness samples of mucosa can be obtained (Figure 13.4).
- Sedation (using xylazine or detomidine combined with butorphanol) is advised to inhibit the cough reflex.
- Diluted local anesthetic solution (injection of 25 to 30mLs of lidocaine diluted with an equal amount of saline)
- 10% formalin and media for bacterial or fungal culture

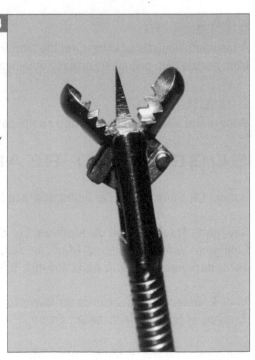

Figure 13.4

A transbronchial lung biopsy is obtained by using an 180cm (or longer) endoscope for horses and a 150cm endoscope for ponies and an endoscopic biopsy forceps that has spikes within or between the biopsy cups to prevent the forceps jaws from sliding.

Procedure

• Diluted local anesthetic solution instilled is administered though the accessory channel or catheter as the scope or catheter is passed to the region of the carina.

• Rarely, disease of the airway mucosa may be grossly visible, and if so, the endoscopic biopsy forceps is advanced to the lesion for biopsy (Figure 13.5).

• An endoscope is passed into a bronchus and wedged. An endoscopic biopsy forceps is advanced into a smaller bronchus until resistance is felt, and then, during inspiration, the forceps is further advanced as far as possible. The jaws of the forceps are opened and then closed.

• Samples are placed in formalin and media for bacterial and fungal culture. A good specimen has a white fluffy appearance and floats. Multiple tissue specimens can be obtained.

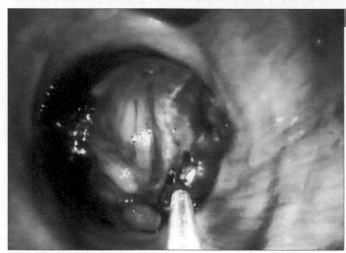

Figure 13.5

Rarely, disease of the airway mucosa may be grossly visible, and if so, the endoscopic biopsy forceps is advanced to the lesion for biopsy.

Interpretation

A histopathologist should interpret the biopsy, but, to our knowledge, histological descriptions of tissue from horses with pulmonary disease obtained by transbronchial lung biopsy have not been reported.

Complications

We are not aware of any reported complications associated with transbronchial lung biopsy.

SUGGESTED READINGS

Raphel CF, Gunson DE. Percutaneous lung biopsy in the horse. *Cornell Veterinarian* 71:439-448, 1981.

Savage C, Traub-Dargatz JL, Mumford EL. Survey of the large animal Diplomates of the American College of Veterinary Internal Medicine regarding percutaneous lung biopsy in the horse *Journal of Veterinary Internal Medicine* 12:456-464, 1998.

Mair T. Diagnostic techniques for lower respiratory tract diseases. In: Robinson, NE ed: *Current Therapy in Equine Medicine 3rd Ed.* pp.299-303, 1992.

Buechner-Maxwell V, Christman M, Murray M, Ley W, Saunders G, Walton A. Transendoscopic biopsy of the horse's airway mucosa. *Journal of Equine Veterinary Science* 16:375-379, 1996.

Chapter 14

COLLECTING URINE

Urine can be collected when the horse urinates or by catheterizating the bladder or ureters.

COLLECTING URINE DURING URINATION

• Most horses, when approached during urination, cease urinating. A collection tube or cup taped to a pole, however, often can be advanced into a urine stream without inhibiting the act of urination (Figure 14.1).
• Palpation of the bladder *per rectum* may give some indication of the likelihood of obtaining voided urine within a reasonable time.

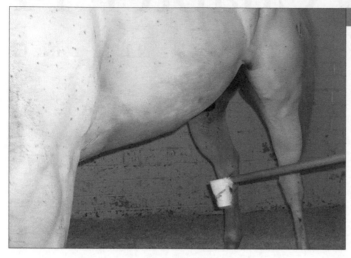

Figure 14.1

A collection tube or cup taped to a pole often can be advanced into a urine stream without inhibiting the act of urination.

• Some horses can be induced to urinate by putting them in a freshly bedded stall.
• Foals usually urinate soon after standing.
• If a catheter is not available for collecting urine, a mare can be stimulated to urinate by digitally palpating its urethra. Many mares urinate within minutes after the finger has been removed from the urethra.
• A plastic gallon jug, with its bottom removed, a collection bag taped to its spout, and straps attached to its base, or an embroidery hoop with a bag attached can be placed over the prepuce and strapped to the back to collect urine from a male horse (Figure 14.2).

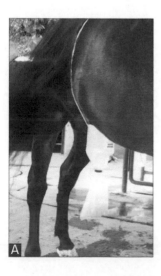
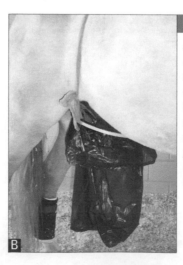

Figure 14.2A & B

A plastic gallon jug, with its bottom removed, a collection bag taped to its spout, and straps attached to its base (A) or an embroidery loop with a bag attached (B), can be placed over the prepuce and strapped to the back for collection of urine.

• **Midstream and end-stream samples** are usually most desirable for cytological examination of urine because nondiagnostic cellular debris is flushed before collection. Cells that have settled out in the bladder, such as neoplastic cells, are found in **an end-stream sample.** Cells indicative of upper urinary tract disease are more likely to be found on a midstream sample, whereas cells indicative of lower urinary tract disease are more likely to be found in an end-stream sample.

• Because urine collected during spontaneous urination contains contaminating bacteria, urine to be submitted for enumeration of pathogenic bacteria should be collected by catheterization.

COLLECTION OF URINE BY CATHETERIZATION OF THE BLADDER (MALE)

Materials
• Having an assistant facilitates catheterization of the male.
• Acepromazine maleate (0.04 mg/kg). Tranquilization facilitates and enhances the safety of the procedure by decreasing resentment of urethral catheterization and by causing relaxation of the retractor penis muscles. When acepromazine is used in stallions (and, rarely, geldings) there is a risk of priapism or penile paralysis that can be minimized by preventing sexual arousal during tranquilization. Sedation using xylazine (0.2 mg/kg) causes diuresis and glucosuria and so may affect results of urinalysis. Although potentially dangerous, urethral catheterization of some horses can be performed without tranquilization.
• The procedure is more safely performed with the horse restrained in stocks.
• A commercially available stallion catheter; or a foal nasogastric tube; or a 30- French, 150-cm long canine feeding tube; or a human enteral feeding tube; or a 100-cm long, 12-mm (or less) diameter endoscope
• A suitable container or a plain glass tube to collect urine
• A sterile, water-soluble lubricant
• Sterile surgical gloves
• Materials for scrubbing the glans penis

Procedure
• The horse is administered a tranquilizer to cause penile protrusion, or alternatively, a hand is inserted through the preputial orifice and the penis is grasped and extracted from the preputial cavity using steady traction.
• An assistant holds and washes the glans with a disinfectant soap.
• The tip of a sterile catheter, dressed with sterile lubricant, is inserted into the urethra, taking care not to insert the catheter tip in the glans fossa. Increased effort may be required to advance the catheter past the ischial arch. As the catheter passes the ischial arch, the horse may raise its tail (i.e., flag) (Figure 14.3). The catheter is inserted about 60cm to reach the bladder.
• Urine may flow spontaneously from the catheter, but if not:
  » A 60-ml catheter tip syringe can be used to apply suction to the tube or to force air through the tube to stimulate the bladder to contract.
  » A hand can be placed in the rectum to compress the bladder.
  » The horse's abdomen can be slapped to cause an abdominal contraction that may cause urine to flow (this, however, may not be a safe method of promoting urine flow from some horses).

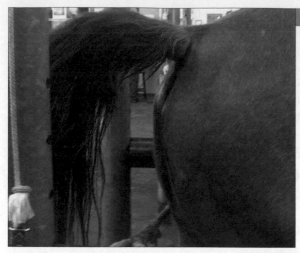

Figure 14.3

As the catheter passes the ischial arch, the horse may raise its tail (i.e., flag).

COLLECTION OF URINE BY CATHETERIZATION OF THE BLADDER (FEMALE)

Materials
- Tranquilization or sedation is optional.
- Tail wrap
- Sterile, water-soluble lubricant
- A rigid, 10- to 14-mm diameter metal or plastic catheter is easiest to pass, but even a flexible Foley or stallion catheter suffices.
- Sterile surgical gloves
- Materials for scrubbing the perineal region

Procedure
- The perineal region is cleaned with a disinfectant soap.
- A lubricated hand is passed into the vestibule, and the urethral opening is identified about 10-cm (knuckle depth) from the labia. A finger is inserted into the urethral opening, and the catheter is advanced beneath the finger *Or* The labia can be spread with fingers, and a lubricated catheter blindly passed along the floor of the vestibule, through the urethra and into the bladder.
- If urine does not flow from the catheter, a hand can be advanced into the vagina, or withdrawn from the vestibule and placed into the rectum, to apply pressure to the bladder.

Complications
- Cystitis is a rare complication, and when it occurs, it is most likely caused by irritation of the bladder mucosa by the catheter during repeated catheterization.
- The urinary catheter may enter an ampulla in a male horse. During palpation of the abdomen *per rectum,* the catheter is felt outside the bladder and is perceived to be free within the abdominal cavity.

COLLECTION OF URINE FROM THE URETERS

Indication

• To localize disease of the urinary tract to one or both kidneys.

Materials

• For male horses, a 100-cm, or longer, endoscope with an outside diameter no greater than 12-mm
• Sterile, polyethylene tubing (Intramedic Polyethylene Tubing, Clay Adams, Becton Dickinson & Co, Parsippany NJ 07054) to fit the accessory channel of the endoscope (e.g., PE 190 tubing for a 9-mm endoscope). Ureteral catheters, to insert into the accessory channel of an endoscope, are commercially available. (Bard USCI polyurethane ureteral catheter, olive tip 5Fr, CR Bard Inc, Murray Hill, NJ; Endoscopic Flushing Catheter, SurgiVet, Waukesha, WI).
• A 10-mL syringe and a hypodermic needle that tightly fits the PE tubing for collection of urine. Sterile, blunt needles that are less likely to cut the PE tubing are commercially available (Monoject Blunt Needles, Sherwood Medical, St. Louis MO 63103).
• Sterile, water-soluble lubricant
• Sterile surgical gloves
• For female horses, a shorter endoscope is adequate. The ureters of mares can also be catheterized blindly using a fairly rigid 8- to 10-Fr polypropylene catheter.
• Materials for scrubbing of the glans penis or perineal region

COLLECTION OF URETERAL URINE USING AN ENDOSCOPE

Procedure

• The insertion tube of the endoscope is passed into the bladder and then withdrawn until the tip of the endoscope lies within the neck of the bladder. The ureteral openings are observed in the dorsal aspect of the trigone region at the 10 and 2 o'clock positions. (The endoscopic view is oriented by observing a pool of urine that is obviously on the floor of the bladder.) Polyethylene tubing is advanced from the biopsy port of the endoscope through the ureteral opening, and urine is aspirated through the tubing (Figure 14.4).

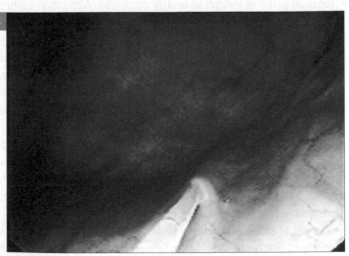

Figure 14.4

To collect urine from a ureter, polyethylene tubing is advanced from the biopsy port of the endoscope through the ureteral opening.

• The ureters of mares can be catheterized blindly, by digitally dilating the urethral orifice to allow introduction of two fingers. The projection of the ureteral orifice is identified by palpation with a fingertip. The finger is withdrawn, and the polyethylene tubing is placed between two fingers, which are reinserted. The urethral orifice is again palpated, and the tubing is threaded into the ureter.

Complications

A ureteral orifice can be difficult to locate. The ureteral openings can be found by watching for dilation of the ureteral orifice as a spurt of urine is discharged. Spurts of urine are discharged about once every minute (Figure 14.5). A ureteral orifice may be easier to see if the bladder is partially distended with air, but too much distention may make an orifice more difficult to see.

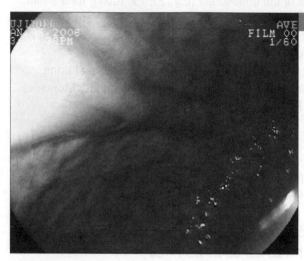

Figure 14.5

The ureteral openings can be found by watching for a spurt of urine that is discharged about once every minute.

URINALYSIS

Interpretation

• If urine cannot be examined within 30 minutes, it should be refrigerated to avoid changes in pH, cellular degeneration, and bacterial growth.
• Urine is first examined for gross appearance, specific gravity, and dipstick reactions, and then centrifuged for microscopic examination of sediment.
• Normal urine is yellow to nearly colorless. Abnormal colors are:
  » **Red to reddish brown:** Normal urine contains *oxidizing agents* that can cause a red or brown discoloration of urine when urine is left standing. This is particularly evident when urine contacts snow. This color is also caused by *hematuria, hemoglobinuria, myoglobinurea,* and *some drugs.* Centrifugation causes urine to clear when hematuria is the cause of red or brown discoloration. Plasma and urine are both discolored red when hemoglobinurea is the cause of reddish discoloration of urine, and concentration of serum creatinine kinase is markedly elevated when myoglobinurea is the cause of discoloration.
  Clear: Indicates dilute urine. Dilute urine is caused by psychogenic water drinking, polydipsia associated with diabetes insipidus or mellitus, fluid therapy, or chronic renal disease.
• Specific gravity is usually *greater than 1.035* (range, 1.020 to 1.060). Urine of foals is very dilute (range, 1.006 or greater). Urinary specific gravity <1.020 in horses with clinical dehydration or azotemia is highly suggestive of renal disease.
• The pH of urine of adult horses is usually *greater than* 8.5, but foals tend to have acidic urine. Prolonged anorexia or a high-grain diet causes the urinary pH to decrease.

- Urine is usually *viscid* because of mucus-secreting cells in the renal pelvis.
- Suspended calcium carbonate crystals cause *opacity* (especially obvious for horses fed a legume hay).
- Small numbers of red blood cells, white blood cells, and bacteria can normally be found in urine sediment. More than 5 RBCs or 5 WBCs per high power field of urine collected midstream during urination or by catheterization is evidence of hemorrhage and inflammation, respectively.
- Recovery of more than 10,000 colony-forming units per mL of urine collected by catheterization is diagnostic of urinary tract infection.
- Dipstick measurement may falsely indicate the presence of protein in highly alkaline urine.
- Granular, cellular, or leukocyte casts indicate renal disease. Hyaline casts can normally be found, especially in urine of exercised horses.
- An increase in urinary concentration of *gamma glutamyltranferase* (UGGT) indicates tubular epithelial necrosis. Comparing the concentration of this urinary enzyme to the concentration of urinary creatinine (Ucr) accounts for the effect of differences in urinary concentration. UGGT/Ucr >50 is evidence of tubular epithelial necrosis.

SUGGESTED READINGS

Schott HC, Hodgson DR, Bayly WM. Ureteral catheterization in the horse. *Equine Veterinary Education* 2:140-143, 1990.

Kohn CW, Chew DJ. Laboratory diagnosis and characterization of renal disease in horses. *The Veterinary Clinics of North America: Equine Practice* 3:585-615, 1987.

Chapter 15

RENAL BIOPSY

Opinions differ concerning the safety of percutaneous renal biopsy. Some clinicians claim that the procedure is safe, even though renal hematoma and hematuria are common complications. Some clinicians, however, consider percutaneous renal biopsy too dangerous for routine use. Fortunately, the use of ultrasonography to examine the kidneys decreases the need for renal biopsy, and when renal biopsy is indicated, ultrasonographic guidance of the biopsy needle may help to avoid complications associated with the procedure. If ultrasonographic equipment is not available, the left kidney is usually biopsied, unless there is evidence that renal disease involves only the right kidney.

RENAL BIOPSY

Indications
- When results of histological examination could influence therapy
- When establishing a prognosis early during the course of disease is important (i.e., is the disease acute and reversible or chronic and irreversible?)
- When a renal mass is found during ultrasonographic examination or during palpation of the left kidney *per rectum*
- To obtain tissue for bacterial culture (e.g., in cases of pyelonephritis)
- To obtain tissue for toxicological study

Contraindications
- Ability of blood to clot should be determined before renal biopsy is performed. The procedure should not be performed on a horse that has a coagulopathy.
- The procedure should not be performed on horses that cannot be adequately restrained or that have tenesmus during palpation *per rectum.* Movement or tenesmus after the biopsy instrument penetrates the body wall can result in laceration of the kidney or spleen.

Materials
- Two clinicians are required to biopsy the left kidney when ultrasonographic equipment is not available.
- Vim-Silverman biopsy needle (See Figure 1.7) or a Tru-Cut style biopsy needle (See Figure 1.4) An automated biopsy instrument (Monopty or Biopty Biopsy Instrument, CR Bard, Inc., Covington GA.) is preferred.
- Sterile surgical gloves and a palpation sleeve
- Fixative (10% formalin) and transport media (or sterile, physiologic saline solution) for bacterial culture
- Local anesthetic solution, a 20-ga., 1.5in. (0.90 x 38 mm) needle, and a #15 or #11 scalpel blade
- Adequate restraint and sedation

Procedure
- Sedation is optional, but restraint should be adequate to prevent movement during the procedure. A lip twitch should be applied.
- **If ultrasonography is not available** the left kidney is usually biopsied. To biopsy the left kidney, feces are removed from the rectum. If the horse is difficult to palpate *per rectum,* epidural anesthesia can be administered, or the rectum can be infused with 50 to100mL of local anesthetic solution. The left paralumbar fossa is prepared for aseptic insertion of the biopsy needle, and skin, at a site on a line connecting the tuber coxae to the point of the shoulder, is anesthetized by subcutaneous injection of 5 to10mL of local anesthetic solution. The exact site for introduction of the biopsy needle can be determined by pushing a finger *per rectum* against the abdominal wall.

• One clinician operates the biopsy instrument while the assistant guides the procedure *per rectum*. A stab incision is made, and the biopsy needle is slowly inserted until it penetrates the peritoneal cavity and can be palpated *per rectum* (Figure 15.1).

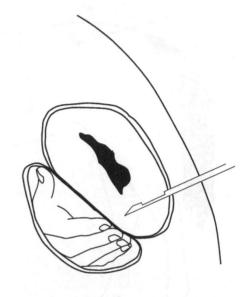

Figure 15.1

For renal biopsy, one clinician operates the biopsy instrument while the assistant guides the procedure per rectum.

• The kidney is then stabilized for insertion of the biopsy needle. The assistant can usually feel the kidney move when the needle enters. An effort should be made to avoid biopsy of the caudal pole of the kidney to avoid major renal vessels. After the needle has contacted the kidney, the biopsy is taken quickly to avoid a laceration that might occur with movement of the horse.

• Three or four samples can be taken and submitted for histological or bacteriological examination. Histological evaluation is improved by taking both a cortical and a medullary sample of kidney. For horses suspected of having glomerulonephritis, some renal tissue can be frozen for immunofluorescence testing.

• **Biopsy following ultrasonographic localization** increases the safety and efficacy of renal biopsy. Using ultrasonography, the right kidney is more easily biopsied. Using ultrasonography, the site of biopsy is identified and the *needle is marked for depth of penetration.*

» The right kidney is biopsied percutaneously usually at the 17th intercostal space, on or above a line connecting the tuber coxae to the point of the shoulder (Figure 15.2) with the needle *inserted perpendicular to the body wall* (Figure 15.3). For most horses, the needle is advanced slightly more than 3 cm to contact the kidney.

» The left kidney is biopsied through the left flank near a line connecting the tuber coxae to the point of the shoulder (Figure 15.4). For some horses, the spleen must be penetrated in order to biopsy the left kidney. Depth of penetration to reach the left kidney is about 7 cm, but this distance varies.

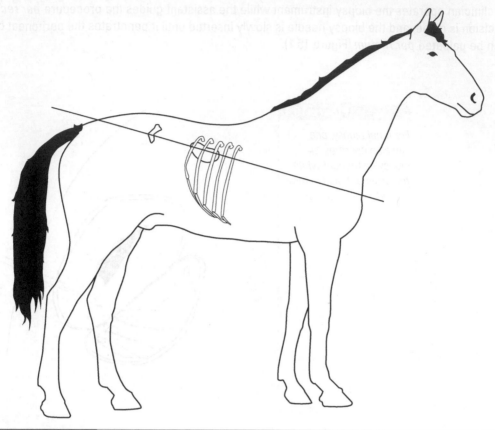

Figure 15.2 *After ultrasonographic localization, the right kidney is biopsied percutaneously usually at the 17th intercostal space on or above a line connecting the tuber coxae to the point of the shoulder.*

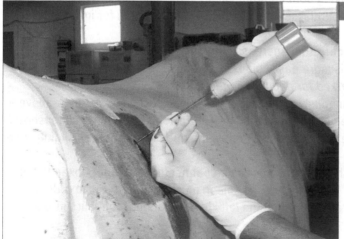

Figure 15.3

The right kidney is biopsied with the needle inserted perpendicular to the body wall. For most horses, the needle is advanced slightly more than 3 cm to contact the kidney.

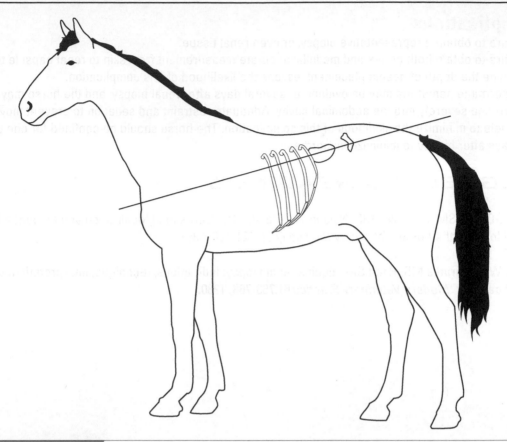

Figure 15.4 *The left kidney is biopsied through the left flank near a line connecting the tuber coxae to the point of the shoulder.*

Interpretation

A histopathologist should interpret the biopsy, but a brief histological description of some renal diseases is presented.

• There is often poor correlation between severity of histological lesions and severity of renal dysfunction in **acute ischemic renal disease** (e.g., some horses with renal failure have very mild histological changes).

• Kidneys of horses with **glomerulonephritis** often have thickened glomerular basement membranes, glomerular hypercellularity, lympho-plasmacytic interstitial nephritis, tubular atrophy and interstitial fibrosis.

• Histologically, **acute pyelonephritis** is characterized by intratubular and interstitial inflammatory cells. Interstitial fibrosis, glomerular atrophy, and loss of tubules and glomeruli are seen in kidneys affected with **chronic pyelonephritis.**

Complications
• Failure to obtain a representative biopsy, or even renal tissue
• Failure to obtain both cortex and medulla; accurate measurement from skin to renal capsule to determine the depth of needle placement lessens the likelihood of this complication.
• Hemorrhage hematuria may be evident for several days after renal biopsy, and the horse may hemorrhage severely into the abdominal cavity. Adequate restraint and sedation to prevent movement help to minimize the likelihood of this complication. The horse should be confined for one to two days after biopsy to minimize hemorrhage.

SUGGESTED READINGS

Barratt-Boyes SM, Spensley MS, Nyland TG, Olander HJ. Ultrasound localization and guidance for renal biopsy in the horse. *Veterinary Radiology* 32: 121-126, 1991.

Bayly WM, Paradis MR, Reed SM. Equine renal biopsy: indications, technique, interpretation, and complications. *Modern Veterinary Practice* 61:763-768, 1980.

Chapter 16

COLLECTION OF ENDOMETRIAL SECRETIONS

Endometrial secretions are collected for cytological examination and for bacterial culture. The greatest value of cytological evaluation of endometrial secretions is in diagnosis of acute endometritis. Secretions for culture and cytology are collected with a guarded sterile swab. Secretions for cytological examination can also be collected by endometrial lavage. The optimal stage of the estrus cycle to collect these secretions is debated, but samples are usually collected when the mare is presented for evaluation, regardless of the stage of the cycle.

COLLECTION OF ENDOMETRIAL SECRETIONS

Indications
- When uterine fluid is detected ultrasonographically during a routine reproductive evaluation
- For mares unexplainably barren
- To determine appropriate uterine therapy when the endometrium is infected
- To determine response to uterine therapy

Contraindications
- **Pregnancy. *The cervix should never be breeched without first determining if the mare is pregnant,*** either by palpating the uterus *per rectum* or by ultrasonographically examining the uterus.
- Maiden mare. Unless uterine fluid is detected ultrasonographically, introduction of a swab may not be worth the slight risk of introducing infection.

COLLECTION OF ENDOMETRIAL SECRETIONS BY LAVAGE

Materials
- The procedure is more safely performed with the mare restrained in stocks.
- Some mares must be restrained with a lip twitch or sedation.
- An obstetrical sleeve and sterile, water-soluble lubrication
- 50mL sterile, physiologic saline solution in a syringe
- A sterile mare infusion (insemination) pipette
- Tail wrap
- A red top, blood collection tube is recommended, but an EDTA tube can be used if endometrial inflammation is severe enough to cause fluid to clot.
- Centrifuge
- Microscope slides

Procedure
- After the mare's perineal region is cleaned with soap and water (some clinicians use only water), a (sterile) gloved, lubricated hand holding an infusion pipette is introduced into the vagina. The index finger is inserted through the cervix, and the pipette is introduced into the cervix along side the finger.
- 50mL sterile, physiologic saline solution is rapidly injected into the uterus and then aspirated by manipulating the tip of the pipette with the finger into different regions of the uterus in search of fluid. Usually, only a small fraction of saline solution is recovered. Manipulation of the uterus *per rectum* may result in recovery of more fluid.

• The aspirated fluid is transferred to collection tubes then centrifuged for 10 minutes. The supernatant is removed, and the cells in the remaining pellet are rolled onto a glass microscope slide with a cotton swab. The slide can be sent to a reference lab for evaluation or stained on site for immediate evaluation.

COLLECTION OF ENDOMETRIAL SECRETIONS WITH A SWAB

Materials
• The procedure is more safely performed with the mare restrained in stocks.
• Some mares must be restrained with a lip twitch or sedation.
• An obstetrical sleeve and sterile, non bacteriocidal/non bacteriostatic, water-soluble lubricant
• Double-guarded endometrial swabs If a double guarded swab is not available, the swab can be double-guarded by passing the single guard containing the swab through a sterile obstetrical sleeve worn over another sterile obstetrical sleeve.
• A transport medium that discourages bacterial growth such as Stuart's or Amies medium is used.
Or:
• Blood agar (and possibly McConkey agar to select for gram negative bacteria), if the swab is to be plated without transport
• Microscope slides for smears for cytologic examination
• A small amount of physiologic saline solution to moisten the swab used to collect secretions for cytology (optional)

Procedure
• After the mare's perineal region is prepared with soap and water (or water alone), a gloved, lubricated hand, holding a guarded endometrial swab (Figure 16.1) is introduced into the vagina. The index finger is inserted through the cervix, and the swab is introduced into the cervix alongside the finger.

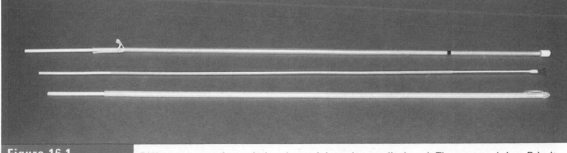

Figure 16.1 *Different types of guarded endometrial swabs are displayed. The top swab is a Priority Care, the middle, a Tiegland, and the bottom, a Kalajian.*

Or:
• If a double-guarded endometrial swab is not available, two sleeves can be worn, and the single-guarded swab is passed between the sleeves along side the index finger, which is inserted through the cervix (Figure 16.2). The single-guarded swab is forced through the finger of the sleeve.
• A swab for culture should be obtained first. If the swab is not immediately streaked onto culture medium, it should be placed in transport medium and refrigerated until it is sent to a laboratory. After swabbing the endometrium for culture, the guard can be left in place, the swab pulled and replaced with another sterile swab pulled from its guard, and the endometrium reswabbed for cytology.

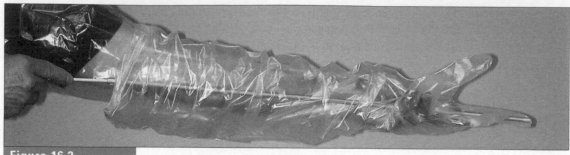

Figure 16.2 *If a guarded endometrial swab is not available, two sleeves can be worn, and the unguarded swab is passed between the sleeves along side the index finger, which is inserted through the cervix.*

- For cytology, moistening a swab with physiologic saline solution improves the quality of the smear (Figure 16.3). The swab must be *gently* rolled on the microscope slide to avoid damaging cells.
- Slides are allowed to air dry.

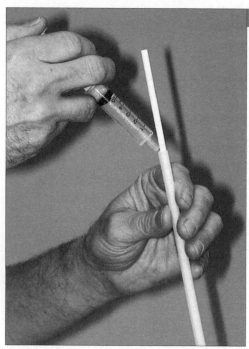

Figure 16.3

For cytology, moistening a swab with physiologic saline solution improves the quality of the smear. To avoid opening the guarded end of the swab, saline can be injected down the lumen of the sleeve.

ENDOMETRIAL CYTOLOGY

Interpretation

- Secretions collected for cytologic evaluation by endometrial lavage may be more representative of endometrial health than are secretions collected with a swab.
- Usually neutrophils are not found during examination of endometrial smears obtained from normal mares (Figure 16.4), and mares with acute endometritis have an obviously large number of neutrophils. More than one neutrophil per 10 epithelial cells or more than 5 neutrophils per high power field (400X) is indicative of endometritis (Figure 16.5).

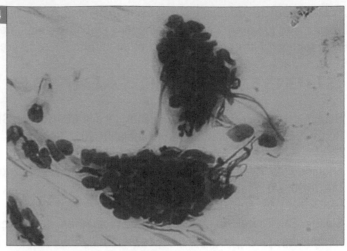

Figure 16.4

Generally, epithelial cells are the only type of cell seen during examination of an endometrial smear of a normal mare. Neutrophils are rarely seen.

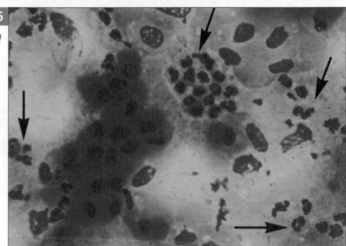

Figure 16.5

More than one neutrophil per 10 epithelial cells is generally considered to be an indication of endometritis. Arrows point to clusters of neutrophils.

• Mares with chronic endometritis may have little evidence of inflammation.

• Epithelial cells range in shape from cuboidal to columnar, and so, finding squamous epithelial cells indicates cervical or vaginal contamination of the swab.

• Eosinophils may be an indication of pneumovagina.

• When results of endometrial cytology do not correlate with results of endometrial culture (i.e., growth of pathogenic bacteria with no neutrophils found during cytologic examination or neutrophils found during cytologic examination with no growth of bacteria), an endometrial biopsy may be necessary to assess the endometrium.

ENDOMETRIAL CULTURE

Interpretation

• Because an endometrial swab is easily contaminated with microorganisms from the vagina, **positive culture results alone should not be used to diagnose endometritis.** Positive culture results should correlate with cytologic or histopathologic evidence of inflammation before infectious endometritis is diagnosed.

• *Streptococcus zooepidemicus, Escherichia coli, Klebsiella pneumonia, Pseudomonas aeruginosa,* yeasts, and fungi are common pathogens that cause endometritis. *Staphylococcus,* alpha-hemolytic streptococci, *Enterobacter sp,* and other enteric bacteria are likely to be contaminants.

SUGGESTED READINGS

Blanchard TL, Varner DD, Schumacher J, Love CC, Brinsko SP, Rigby SL. Manual of Equine Reproduction. 2nd ed. Mosby, Philadelphia, 2002, 253 pages.

England CW. Allen's Fertility and Obstetrics in the Horse, 2nd ed. Blackwell Science, Cambridge, MA, 1996, 241 pages.

Slusher SH, Cowell RL, Tyler RD. The endometrium. In: Cowell, RL, Tyler RD. eds. Cytology and Hematology of the Horse. American Veterinary Publications, Inc., Goleta, CA, 1992, pp.173-190.

Pycock J. Pre-breeding checks for mares. In Practice, Vol. 26:78-85, 2004.

Chapter 17

ENDOMETRIAL BIOPSY

Histologic examination of the endometrium is valuable in detecting or confirming chronic disease of the endometrium and predicting the potential fertility of a mare. Endometrium can be safely biopsied during any stage of the mare's cycle, but there is less chance of error in predicting fertility when biopsies from diestral mares are interpreted. To be of value, endometrial biopsies should be evaluated by clinicians or pathologists experienced at examining such specimens.

ENDOMETRIAL BIOPSY

Indications
- For diagnosis of uterine abnormalities detected during palpation *per rectum* or ultrasonographic examination
- For repeat breeders (i.e., mares with more than 3 returns to service during the same breeding season)
- For mares that have aborted (For accurate interpretation, it is best to wait about 6 weeks after an abortion before an endometrial biopsy is taken.)
- For non-pregnant mares that are not cycling during the physiologic breeding season
- For mares requiring urogenital surgery (Urogenital surgery may not be economically justified for some mares with extensive endometrial disease.)
- For mares unexplainably barren
- For mares with pyometra
- Rarely, as part of a routine reproductive examination

Contraindications
- **Pregnancy. *The cervix should never be breached until the mare is determined not to be pregnant*** by palpating or ultrasonographically examining the uterus per rectum.

Materials
- An alligator-type endometrial forceps, at least 70 cm long with a 20- x 4-x 3-mm basket, is recommended (Figure 17.1). (Samples smaller than 20 mm may be inadequate for reliable interpretation.)
- An obstetrical sleeve and sterile, water-soluble lubrication
- A small gauge, hypodermic needle for removal of the tissue sample from the forceps
- 10% buffered formalin or Bouin's solution. Some pathologists have a definite preference for specimens fixed with one of these solutions. Tissue fixed in Bouin's solution for more than 24 hours, may become brittle and difficult to section, and stain poorly with hematoxylin. Endometrial tissue should be transferred to formalin before transport. (Alternatively, samples arriving in Bouin's solution can be placed in 70% alcohol for softening before sectioning.)

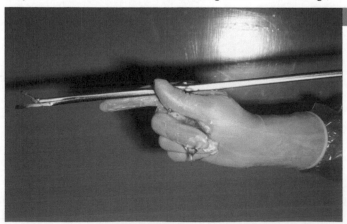

Figure 17.1

An alligator-type forceps at least 70 cm long with a 20- x 4-x 3-mm basket is recommended for endometrial biopsy.

• The biopsy forceps can be cold sterilized when samples from more than one mare are to be taken, or when sterilizing the forceps with heat is impractical. A cold-sterilized forceps should be rinsed with sterile water or physiologic saline solution before use. A capped, 80-cm, 1-in PVC pipe makes a convenient container for the disinfectant (Figure 17.2).

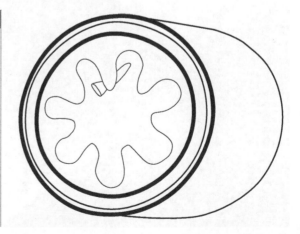

Figure 17.2

A capped, 80-cm, 1-in PVC pipe makes a convenient container for storing the endometrial biopsy rod in disinfectant.

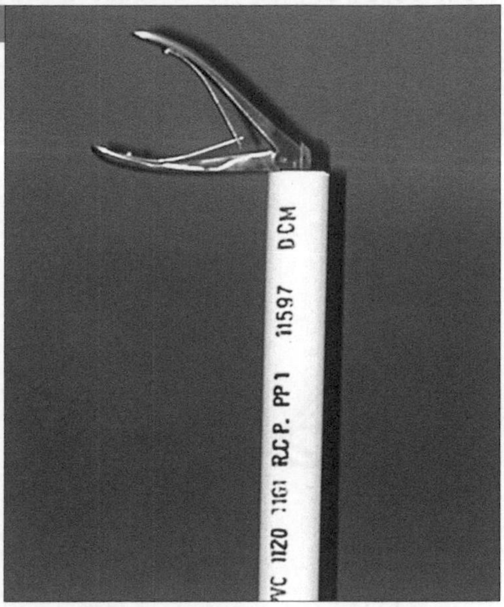

Procedure

• *The mare is determined not to be pregnant by palpating or ultrasonographically examining the uterus* per rectum.
• Restraint for biopsy is the same as for safe palpation *per rectum.* The tail is wrapped or held to the side, and the external genitalia are cleaned. Endometrial swabs for bacterial culture and cytologic examination always are obtained before biopsy.
• The biopsy forceps, with the jaws closed, is carried along side the gloved index finger through the cervix. **At this point two alternative techniques are possible.**
• With gentle probing, the forceps basket can be maneuvered 7 to 10 cm into the uterus. The jaws are opened and then blindly closed over a fold of endometrium (Figure 17.3), and the sample is removed with a sharp tug. The mare generally displays no signs of discomfort when the tissue is removed. **Or:**

Figure 17.3

One method of endometrial biopsy is to maneuver the biopsy instrument into the uterine lumen. The jaws are then opened and closed over a natural uterine fold.

• The hand is removed from the vagina and placed into the previously emptied rectum. The forceps is turned on its side, the jaws are opened, and a finger is pressed down until it can be felt between the jaws. The jaws are closed and the sample is removed with a sharp tug (Figure 17.4). This method allows more accurate placement of the forceps. Also, endometrium must be pushed into the jaws of the forceps if air has been introduced into the uterus, because air in the uterus causes the folds of endometrium to disappear.

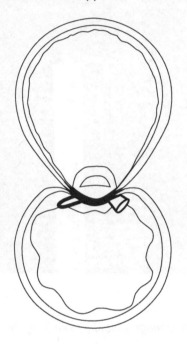

Figure 17.4

By placing a hand in the rectum and pushing endometium into the jaws of the biopsy instrument, endometrium can be obtained when air in the uterus has caused the natural folds to disappear.

• The sample should be removed from the basket of the forceps with a small hypodermic needle and placed in a fixative (Figure 17.5).
• One sample is *usually* representative of the entire endometrium, but a biopsy taken from the usual site of embryonic fixation (i.e., the junction between body and horn) is most likely to provide accurate information. If there is a specific area of interest previously identified during palpation *per rectum,* or during ultrasonographic or endoscopic examination of the uterus, the biopsy should be taken from that site.

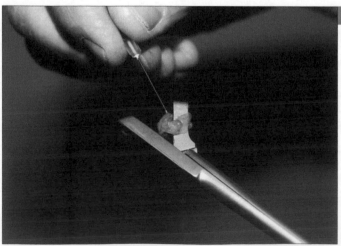

Figure 17.5

To avoid creation of histological artifacts, the tissue sample should be removed from the basket of the forceps with a small hypodermic needle.

Complications

• If care is taken to avoid procuring an endometrial biopsy from a pregnant mare, this procedure is safe. The endometrium of mares can be repeatedly biopsied without affecting fertility.

• Although it is not necessarily a complication, the clinician should be aware that some mares that are biopsied during the midleuteal phase of their cycle might experience a shortened diestrus. The endometrial trauma or transient infection associated biopsy can induce a release of $PGF_2\alpha$ to cause luteolysis.

Interpretation

A pathologist or clinician experienced at interpreting endometrial, microscopic anatomy should examine the biopsy. Pathologic changes indicate the chronicity of disease.

• Infiltration of the luminal epithelium and stroma with neutrophils indicates acute endometritis.

• Fungi appear black or gray when stained with a silver stain such as Gomori's methanamine silver stain.

• Infiltration of the stroma with mononuclear cells (i.e., lymphocytes, plasma cells, and macrophages) indicates chronic endometritis.

• Diffuse or periglandular fibrosis with dilated lymphatics indicates chronic endometritis.

• Glandular inactivity and luminal epithelial cells unresponsive to hormonal influences indicate endometrial atrophy.

The endometrial biopsy is categorized according to endometrial changes that indicate the mare's ability to carry a foal to term. Several different endometrial scoring systems have been published. Kenny's (one of the most commonly used) scoring scale is:

• Category I: Normal endometrium. 70%, or greater, chance to carry a foal to term.

• Category IIA: Mild changes generally associated with infiltration of inflammatory cells. 50-70% chance to carry a foal to term.

• Category IIB: Moderate changes generally associated with fibrosis. 30-50% chance to carry a foal to term.

• Category III: Severe, irreversible changes that interfere with ability to conceive and carry a foal to term. These mares have less than a 10% chance of conceiving and carrying a foal to term.

SUGGESTED READINGS

Carleton CL. Clinical examination of the non-pregnant female reproductive tract. In: *Current Therapy In Large Animal Theriogenology,* Ed: Younquist, RS. WB Saunders Co. 1997, pp. 79-95.

Blanchard TL, Varner DD, Schumacher J, Love CC, Brinsko SP, Rigby SL. *Manual of Equine Reproduction.* 2nd ed. Mosby. Philadelphia. 2002, 253 pages.

England CW. *Allen's Fertility and Obstetrics in the Horse, 2nd ed.* Blackwell Science, Cambridge, MA, 1996, 241 pages.

Chapter 18

COLLECTION OF SEMEN

Semen can be collected in an artificial vagina or in a condom. Semen collected in a condom is inferior in quality because it is contaminated with debris from the penis. Depending on the temperament and training of the stallion, the receptivity of the jump mare, and experience of personnel, collection of semen can be a dangerous and, sometimes, a very frustrating procedure.

COLLECTION OF SEMEN

Indications
• As part of a breeding soundness examination
• For artificial insemination

COLLECTION OF SEMEN WITH AN ARTIFICIAL VAGINA

Materials
• At least three people are required if a mare, rather than a phantom, is used as a mount-- a handler for the stallion, a handler for the mare, and the collector.
• An artificial vagina (AV). Many models are commercially available each having advantages and disadvantages. Commonly used models include the Missouri (NASCO, Fort Atkinson WI.), Colorado [and modified versions of the Colorado, the CSU (Animal Reproduction Systems, Chino CA.) and Lane (Lane Manufacturing, Denver, CO.) models], and the Japanese (Nishikawa) (Figure 18.1). The Missouri AV is

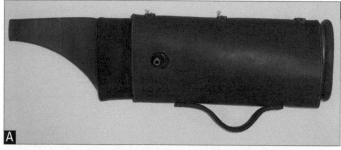

Figure 18.1A, B & C

Some of the commercially available artificial vaginas are displayed, the (A) Missouri, (B) Nishikawa, and (C) Colorado Models.

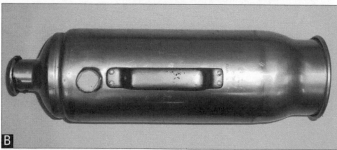

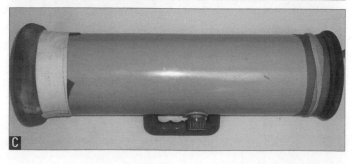

popular because it is lightweight and inexpensive. For stallions that prefer a very warm AV, the temperature of the inner lining of the Missouri AV can be increased without damaging spermatozoa, because the ejaculate is less likely to contact the lining of the water jacket.

• Water warmed to 48° to 50° C (118° to122° F) to fill the water jacket of the AV to achieve a temperature in the liner of 44° to 48° C (112° to 118° F). For AVs that collect the ejaculate with minimal exposure of the ejaculate to the liner, such as the Missouri AV, the water jacket can be filled with water heated to create a temperature of 48° to 55° C (118° to 131° F) in the liner. A thermometer taped to the water faucet allows the water temperature to be adjusted, so that water flows from the faucet into the AV at the desired temperature (Figure 18.2).

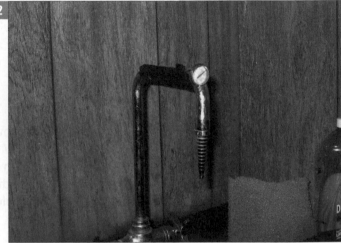

Figure 18.2

A thermometer taped to the water faucet allows the water temperature to be adjusted, so that water flows from the faucet into the artificial vagina at the desired temperature.

• Commercially available disposable liners for the AV (Har-Vet, Spring Valley WI.) (optional) (Figure 18.3). Or, use a rubber liner that has been cleaned with tap water only (to avoid spermicidal soap residues), rinsed with distilled water and disinfected by submerging it in ethyl or isopropyl alcohol and then allowed to air-dry before use.

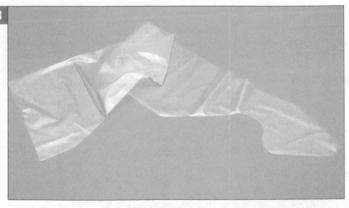

Figure 18.3

Commercially available disposable liners for the artificial vagina minimize clean up.

• Filters to attach to the AV to trap the gel fraction of the ejaculate as it flows to the collection bottle. Polyester filters made from inline milk filters (NASCO, Fort Atkinson WI.) trap more sperm than do nylon mesh microfilters (Animal Reproduction Systems, Chino, CA.) (Figure 18.4). For reuse, the nylon filters can be rinsed first in tap water, then in distilled water, then disinfected by submersion in ethyl or isopropyl alcohol, and then air-dried.

• An obstetrical sleeve

• Sterile, non-spermicidal lubricating jelly

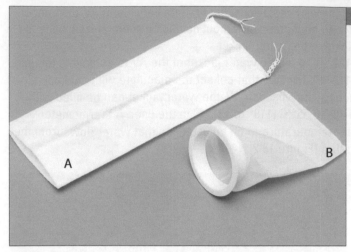

Figure 18.4

Polyester filters (A) made from inline milk filters trap more sperm than do nylon mesh microfilters (B).

• A receptive mare (i.e., one in estrus or one that has been ovariectomized) or a phantom (dummy) mount. Many stallions readily thrust and ejaculate into an AV without a mount (i.e., ground collection) if a mount is not available, or if the stallion has not been trained to mount a phantom (Figure 18.5). Hobbles and a lip twitch applied to the mare increase the safety of the stallion and personnel during collection of semen (Figure 18.6). The mare's tail should be wrapped to prevent tail hairs from entering the AV and lacerating the penis.
• Safety helmets for personnel
• A chain shank to restrain the stallion
• Cotton soaked in warm water. A mild, non-disinfectant soap, can be used to clean the stallion's penis and the mare's perineum (optional).
• An incubator to maintain the temperature of all glassware or other equipment that contacts the ejaculate at 37° to 39° C (99 °to 102° F)

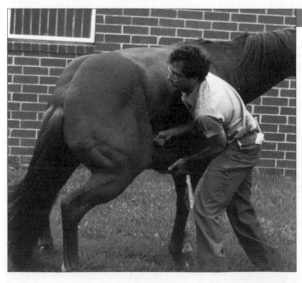

Figure 18.5

Even without a mount, many stallions readily thrust and ejaculate into an artificial vagina. To increase the safety of collection some clinicians prefer to use a helmet.

Figure 18.6A & B

*Hobbles and a lip twitch applied to the mare increase the safety of the stallion and personnel during collection of semen. The rear limbs (**A**) or a front limb (**B**) can be hobbled.*

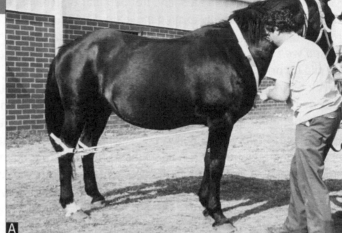
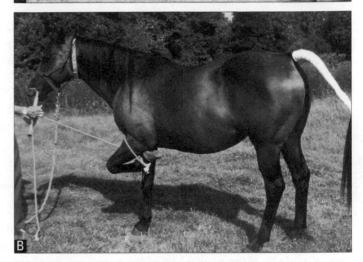

Procedure

• The AV is prepared at the desired temperature, and warm, sterile, lubricating jelly is applied to the proximal portion of the liner using an obstetrical sleeve. To prevent debris from entering the lumen of the AV, the sleeve is left in the AV and reflected over its opening until the AV is ready for use (Figure 18.7).

Figure 18.7

To prevent debris from entering the lumen of the artificial vagina, the sleeve is left in the artificial vagina and reflected over its opening until the artificial vagina is ready for use.

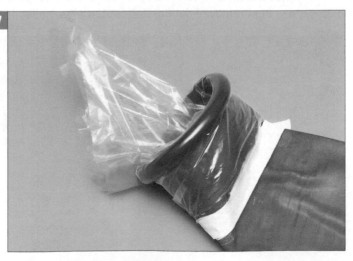

- The mare's tail is wrapped, and her perineal region and hindquarters are cleaned.
- The stallion is sexually excited at a safe distance from the mare, and debris from the penis is removed with warm water [about 42° C (108° F)], and cotton. *If soap is used, the penis should be rinsed well to avoid contact of the ejaculate with soap because soap is spermicidal.* The penis should be dried prior to collecting semen.
- The restrained mare (or phantom) is approached at a wide angle from the left, and the stallion is introduced to the mare's left shoulder. The stallion is allowed to slowly work his way back to the mare's hindquarters. If the mare appears receptive, and if the stallion has at least a partial erection, the stallion is allowed to mount. The stallion handler can grasp the stallion's left forelimb, as the stallion begins to thrust, to support the stallion and to protect the collector.
- The penis is deflected (not grasped and shoved) into the AV, which is held with the left hand at the mare's hip, parallel to the body of the mare and at the level of the vulva. The AV is maintained in this position during thrusting. Forcing the artificial vagina against the mare's hip minimizes movement of the AV, caused by thrusting of the stallion (Figure 18.8).

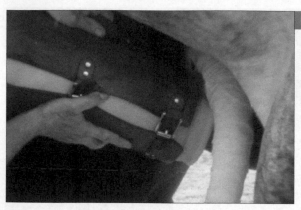

Figure 18.8

Forcing the artificial vagina against the mare's hip minimizes movement of the artificial vagina, caused by thrusting of the stallion.

- The receptacle end of the AV is lowered soon after the stallion begins to ejaculate. Ejaculation is signaled by cessation of thrusting, by urethral pulsations, which can be felt by holding fingers on the ventral surface of the caudal part of the penis, and by observing the stallion to "flag" (i.e., to raise and lower its tail).
- The ejaculate should be protected from adverse conditions, such as light, cold, or excessive heat. If gel was not filtered during collection, it can be removed by pouring the ejaculate through a filter. Or gel can be removed by aspirating a strand of it into a 60-ml syringe and then gently lifting the gel from the ejaculate, while continuing to aspirate the gel (Figure 18.9). To minimize loss of spermatozoa, gel is best removed during, rather than after, collection.

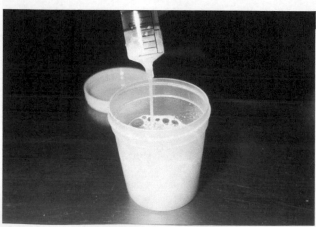

Figure 18.9

Gel can be removed by aspirating a strand of gel into a 60-ml syringe and then gently lifting the gel from the ejaculate, while continuing to aspirate the gel. To minimize loss of spermatozoa, gel is best removed during, rather than after, collection.

COLLECTING SEMEN WITH A CONDOM

Materials

• Three people are required to collect semen with a condom-the mare handler, the stallion handler, and the collector.

• A commercial stallion condom (Har-Vet, Spring Valley WI.) or a latex surgical glove (Figure 18.10) If a surgical glove is used, it should be thoroughly rinsed with water, to remove all traces of powder, and dried, because water is spermicidal. Some gloves may be spermicidal, and this should be determined before collecting semen for evaluation or for breeding.

• A large, stout rubber band

• Water soluble, sterile, non-spermicidal lubricating jelly

• Safety helmets for personnel

• A chain shank for restraint of the stallion

• Cotton soaked in warm water a mild, non-disinfectant soap can be used for cleaning the stallion's penis (optional).

• An incubator to maintain all glassware or other equipment, which contacts the ejaculate, at 37° to 39° C (99° to 102° F)

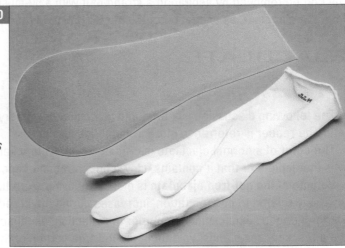

Figure 18.10

A commercial stallion condom or a latex surgical glove can be used to collect stallion semen. Semen collected in a condom is inferior in quality because it is contaminated with debris from the penis.

Procedure

• The stallion is sexually excited at a safe distance from the mount, and smegma is removed from the penis with warm water [about 42° C (108° F)], and cotton. If soap is used, it should be completely rinsed off. The penis should be dried, before the condom is applied.

• If the stallion does not lose its erection during washing, the condom or glove can be applied at this time, or the stallion can again be sexually stimulated to cause an erection.

• The condom is placed over the glans penis and secured with the rubber band. Most stallions do not object to placement of the rubber band. It is important to force all air from the condom after it is applied to the penis (Figure 18.11).

• The condom is generously coated with lubricating jelly.

• The restrained mare is approached at a wide angle from the left, and the stallion is introduced to the mare at the mare's left shoulder. The stallion is allowed to slowly work its way back to the mare's hindquarters. If the mare appears receptive, and if the stallion has at least a partial erection, the stallion is allowed to mount. The stallion handler can grasp the stallion's left forelimb, as the stallion begins to thrust, to give the stallion more support and to protect the collector.

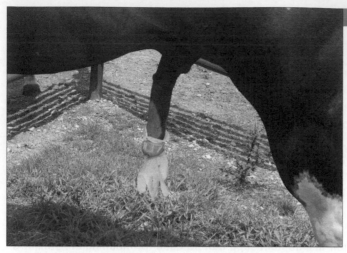

Figure 18.11

The condom or glove is placed over the glans penis and secured with a rubber band. Most stallions do not object to placement of the rubber band.

- The collector places a hand at the top of the labia to deflect the penis into the vagina.
- As soon as the stallion dismounts after ejaculation, the rubber band and condom are removed.
- The ejaculate should be protected from adverse conditions, such a light, cold or excessive heat. Gel can be removed by aspirating a strand of it with a 60-ml syringe and then gently lifting the gel from the ejaculate, as aspiration of the gel is continued (See Figure 18.9).

EJACULATE

Interpretation

- The following discussion is a brief and incomplete summary concerning evaluation of the ejaculate. The reader is referred to more in-depth discussions.
- **The color** of a normal ejaculate is creamy white; watery semen is an indication that the ejaculate was incomplete or that it contains a low concentration of spermatozoa.
- **Volume of the gel-free ejaculate** is measured using a graduated cylinder. Volume, which is inversely related to concentration, increases during the breeding season. Volume also increases with prolonged sexual stimulation prior to collection, because of an increase in fluid produced by the accessory sex glands. Volume of the gel-free portion of the ejaculate has little influence on fertility; a large volume of semen may slightly decrease fertility, however, because a portion of a large ejaculate may be expelled from the uterus.
- **Spermatozoal motility** of the gel-free portion of the ejaculate is usually evaluated subjectively on a slide warmed to 37° or 38° at 200x magnification, using a light microscope. Overall motility usually ranges from 60 to 80%, and progressive motility ranges from 40 to 60%. If the ejaculate is to be diluted with an extender and used for breeding, it is wise to examine sperm motility of the ejaculate mixed (1 to 20) with the extender. A skim milk-glucose extender (E-Z Mixin Equine Semen Extender, Animal Reproduction Systems, 14395 Ramona Ave., Chino CA. 91710, 800-300-5143, or mix 2L of 5% dextrose with one, 24g packet of dry, nonfat milk) is commonly used for this purpose. Sperm motility is easier to assess in an extended sample.
- **Longevity of sperm motility** is determined using raw semen stored at room temperature (20 to 25 C°) and using semen diluted in extender stored at room temperature or refrigerated (4 to 6 C°). Results provide a *rough* estimation of the ability of the sperm to survive in the mare's reproductive tract. There are no established criteria for reference when performing this test, but stallions having very short sperm longevity can be identified. Raw semen from fertile stallions should maintain at least 10% progressive motility for 6 hours at room temperature. Semen of stallions, whose sperm

cools well, has very little deterioration in total and progressive motility after 24 hours of storage at 5 C°. Semen initially having good sperm motility that quickly deteriorates should be reexamined using a different extender. The Society of Theriogenology guidelines for evaluating the semen of prospective breeding stallions recommends that, for semen samples maintained in a light-shielded environment, at least 10% progressive motile sperm should be present in raw and extended semen for 6 and 24 hours, respectively.

• A normal ejaculate of a stallion contains at least 60% morphologically normal sperm. The number of morphologically *normal* sperm is more important than the number of morphologically *abnormal* sperm. **Sperm morphology** is assessed by examining air-dried slides of semen stained with Hancock's stain using a 3:2 semen-to-stain ratio. The morphology of 100 sperm from the ejaculate is examined at 1000x magnification. Dead sperm stain red ("red is dead"). Sperm defects that include malformed heads, midpieces, or tails, and abnormalities of the acrosome are associated with spermatogenesis and are more likely to be associated with decreased fertility (Figure 18.12). Sperm defects such kinked tails or midpieces, detached heads, and cytoplasmic droplets occur during tubular transport or are caused by poor semen handling techniques and have little effect on fertility (Figure 18.13).

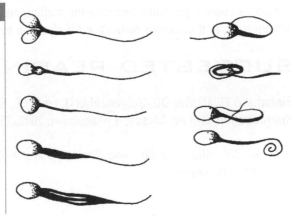

Figure 18.12

Sperm defects such as malformed heads, midpieces, or tails, are associated with spermatogenesis and are more likely to be associated with decreased fertility.

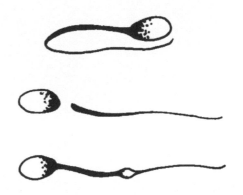

Figure 18.13

Sperm defects that occur during tubular transport or are caused by poor semen handling techniques include kinked tails, detached heads, and cytoplasmic droplets. These defects have little effect on fertility.

- **Concentration of spermatozoa** in the gel-free portion of the ejaculate is determined using a hemocytometer or a hemocytometer-calibrated spectrophotometer or densiometer. By multiplying spermatozoal concentration times the volume of the gel-free portion of the ejaculate, the **total spermatozoa per ejaculate** are determined. A minimum insemination dose of at least 100 million progressively motile spermatozoa is recommended for breeding efficiency in an artificial insemination program. An increase in fertility is not observed by using more than 500 million progressively motile spermatozoa per insemination.
- The **pH** of normal stallion semen ranges from 7.2 to 7.6, but begins to decrease soon after collection. A high pH may indicate that the ejaculate is contaminated with urine or that the accessory sex glands are infected. pH can be measured using a pH meter (Digital Ionalyzer, Orion Research, Cambridge, MA) or litmus paper that is sensitive enough to indicate 0.1 increments in pH.

Complications

- Injury of personnel or the stallion; using trained personnel for the procedure minimizes danger of injury. Use of a phantom, rather than a mare, for mounting greatly decreases the risk of injury for personnel as well as for the stallion.
- Failure to obtain an ejaculate; after 3 or 4 fruitless attempts at collection, the stallion should be returned to its stall for several hours. When the procedure is repeated later, a new jump mare should be used, if possible, because the stallion may have an aversion to the original mare. The temperature and pressure within the AV also can be changed. Some stallions prefer a very hot AV.

SUGGESTED READINGS

Blanchard TL, Varner DD, Schumacher J, Love CC, Brinsko SP, Rigby SL. *Manual of Equine Reproduction, 2nd ed.* Mosby, Philadelphia, 2002, 253 pages.

England CW. *Allen's Fertility and Obstetrics in the Horse, 2nd ed.* Blackwell Science, Cambridge, MA, 1996, 241 pages.

Chapter 19

TESTICULAR BIOPSY

The testes of horses are infrequently biopsied because reports of the procedure in other species often cite complications. Reports of complications associated with split needle or aspiration biopsies of the equine testis, however, are rare. A **fine needle aspiration biopsy** is the least invasive but may produce a sample that is too small for diagnosis. The **incisional or open biopsy technique** provides the largest sample and direct visualization of the testicular vasculature, but it is also the most invasive technique and has a higher incidence of complication. The most commonly used technique for testicular biopsy is the **split needle method,** which usually provides adequate tissue for a diagnosis and is unlikely to have deleterious effects. With ultrasonographic guidance, the split needle technique is also useful for biopsying small discrete lesions.

TESTICULAR BIOPSY

Indications
• When less invasive methods have failed to supply an etiologic or pathologic diagnosis that is essential to determine treatment and prognosis of infertility or subfertility in stallions
• For diagnosis of discrete, nodular lesions
• When horses with chronically enlarged testes have not responded to anti-inflammatory and antimicrobial therapy
• When neoplasia is suspected but can not be diagnosed or ruled out using less invasive techniques

Contraindications
• Known testicular tumors. The procedure may increase dissemination of neoplastic cells. A neoplastic testis should be surgically removed with as much of the spermatic cord and parietal tunic, as possible.
• Any condition that can be diagnosed by non-invasive means
• Although complications of testicular biopsy such as infection and fibrosis are unlikely, the procedure should be performed only after exhausting other diagnostic techniques.

ASPIRATION BIOPSY

Materials
• 5- or12-mL syringe
• Microscope slides
• Sedation and a lip twitch
• 20-ga. (0.90 mm) hypodermic needle

Procedure
• Performed with the horse standing, sedated and twitched
• The 20-ga needle is inserted through the scrotal skin into the testicular parenchyma, and the syringe is attached.
• The plunger is withdrawn to create suction, and while maintaining suction, the needle is directed to several different areas of testicular parenchyma.
• The plunger is gently released before removing the needle from the parenchyma.
• Digital pressure over the puncture site for several minutes may decrease the likelihood of hematoma formation.
• Aspirated material is expelled onto slides and gently smeared (cells are extremely fragile).

SPLIT NEEDLE BIOPSY

Materials

- #15 blade and sterile surgical gloves
- Sedation and a lip twitch
- 2-3 mL mepivacaine HCl
- A 12- or 14-ga, automated biopsy needle (Monopty or Biopty Biopsy Instrument, CR Bard, Inc., Covington GA. These needles have a penetration depth of 22 mm) or a manually operated, 12- or 14-ga Vim-Silverman or Tru-Cut style biopsy needle.
- Bouin's solution (the fixative of choice, because it causes the least tissue shrinkage and provides the greatest nuclear detail) (Figure 19.1). Formalin is a less desirable fixative, because it causes tissue shrinkage and a loss of structural detail, provides poor nuclear images, and can result in the loss of mature spermatozoa.

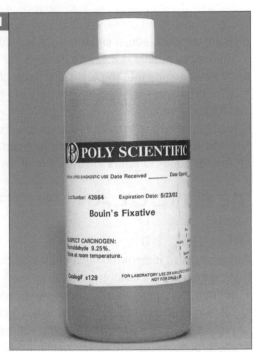

Figure 19.1

Bouin's solution is the fixative of choice for testicular tissue because it causes the least tissue shrinkage and provides the greatest nuclear detail.

Procedure

- Performed with the horse standing or anesthetized
- The scrotum is surgically prepared
- Unless there is a particular area of interest, the point of entry for the biopsy needle is the antero-lateral portion of the testis, away from the head of the epididymis (Figure 19.2) where surface vasculature is least prominent. To sample a discrete lesion, ultrasonography may be needed to guide the needle to obtain a representative biopsy.
- After scrubbing the scrotal skin, the skin and subcutaneous tissue is infiltrated with a local anesthetic solution using a 23- to 25-ga (0.65- to 0.5-mm) hypodermic needle. Anesthetic solution should not be placed within the testis. Doing so could cause bleeding that could interfere with interpretation of the biopsy or induce testicular degeneration.

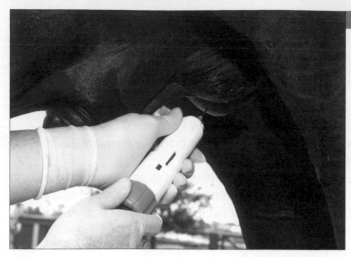

Figure 19.2

*Unless there is a partic-
ular area of interest, the
point of entry for the
biopsy needle is the
anterolateral portion of
the testis, away from the
head of the epididymis.*

• Using the #15 blade, a small incision is made through the skin, which is held tense against the testis.
• The biopsy needle is inserted through the incision and forced through the vaginal tunics and tunica albuguinea into the testicular parenchyma.
• After the biopsy is removed, the tissue is gently teased off the instrument into the fixative using a small gauge needle.
• A single suture is usually adequate to close the scrotal skin.
• Testicular biopsy samples should be fixed for about 12 hours in Bouin's solution, washed and stored for about 12 hours in 70% ethanol, and then stored or shipped to a laboratory in 50% ethanol.

TESTICULAR BIOPSY

Interpretation

A reproductive histopathologist should study the biopsy, but a brief histological description of some testicular diseases or interpretation of the findings is presented.
• Inflammatory cellular infiltrates are an indication of bacterial orchitis.
• Cytological examination of a testicular aspirate will not provide details concerning testicular organization but may provide a crude estimate of germ cell numbers and identify inflammatory cells.
• The prognosis for fertility for stallions with low numbers of sperm that have abnormal germinal epithelium (i.e., stallions with testicular degeneration) depends on the degree of germinal damage. Semen quality of some stallions with mild testicular degeneration may eventually improve.
• Stallions with low numbers of sperm that have normal germinal epithelium should be examined for blockage of spermatozoal transport.

Complications

• **Scrotal edema** that disappears within 5 days
• **Intra-testicular hemorrhage,** with possible damage of the parenchyma, caused by pressure necrosis
• **Possible immune reaction to spermatozoa** caused by disruption of the blood-testis barrier
In one study, however, antisperm antibodies were not detected in serum or seminal plasma of stallions subsequent to testicular biopsy.
• Possible dissemination of neoplastic cells, if a tumor is biopsied

• A transient decrease in semen quality after testicular biopsy is reported in other species, but is not reported for the horse.

• Formation of a hematoma between the testicular tissue and the tunics, or between the tunics and scrotum, is the most common complication and can result in insulation-induced damage to the seminiferous epithelium. Gentle handling of the testis during biopsy and procurement of the specimen from the recommended location can minimize hematoma formation. Gently pinching the incision site with a sterile sponge after the biopsy is taken may be beneficial in preventing hemorrhage.

SUGGESTED READINGS

Threlfall WR, Lopate C. Testicular biopsy. In: McKinnon AO, Voss JL, eds. *Equine Reproduction.* Lea & Febiger, 1993, pp. 943-949.

Dascanio JJ. Examination of the scrotum, testis, prepuce, and penis. In Wolfe DF, Moll HD, eds: Large Animal Urogenital Surgery. Williams & Wilkins, 1999, pp. 17-21.

Faber NF, Rosner JF. Testicular biopsy in stallions: diagnostic potential and effects on prospective fertility. Journal of Reproduction and Fertility Supplement 56:31-42, 2000.

Chapter 20

ABDOMINOCENTESIS

(PERITONEAL TAP)

Peritoneal fluid is commonly collected and analyzed to aid in evaluating horses with abdominal disease. Many abdominal diseases can be diagnosed by cytological examination of peritoneal fluid.

ABDOMINOCENTESIS

Indications
- For some horses with signs of acute abdominal pain (i.e., when physical examination alone does not supply enough information to determine a course of action)
- For horses with recurrent signs of abdominal pain
- For horses with unexplainable weight-loss
- For foals with suspected rupture of the bladder
- For horses with chronic diarrhea
- For horses with suspected abdominal neoplasia (e.g., when masses are felt during palpation of the abdomen *per rectum,* or when the horse has an unexplained increase in seruminal concentration of globulin)

Contraindications
- When results will not influence case management (e.g., a horse scheduled for exploratory celiotomy regardless of the results of analysis of peritoneal fluid)
- When there is a large amount of markedly distended small intestine, risk versus benefit should be considered, because accidental puncture of small intestine may result in a continual leak of intestinal fluid as long as the intestine remains distended.

Materials
- An 18- or 19-ga (1.2- or 1.1-mm) needle. For most horses, a 1.5-in (3.8-cm) hypodermic needle will suffice, but for fat horses, a 3.5-in (8.89 cm) spinal needle may be necessary to reach the abdominal cavity. **Or:**
- Sterile surgical gloves, a #11 or #15 scalpel blade, a 3.5-in (8.89 cm) teat cannula or a bitch catheter, a pledget of cotton or a gauze sponge, and 2 to 3mL of local anesthetic solution.
- Collection tubes (a tube containing EDTA and a clot tube).

Procedure
- Some horses require a lip twitch and local anesthesia of the skin at the site of centesis. Horses with acute abdominal pain often require little restraint and no local anesthesia at the site of centesis. Foals requiring abdominocentesis always should be maximally restrained.
- The site of centesis can be determined ultrasonographically by finding a region where fluid has collected. The usual site of centesis is at the midline at the most dependent area between the xyphoid and the umbilicus. Some clinicians prefer to perform abdominocentesis at a site far behind the umbilicus. Abdominocentesis can be performed at a site off the midline, but, away from the midline, fat lining the abdominal cavity may be so thick that a 1.5 inch needle will not reach the abdominal cavity.
- **If a hypodermic needle is used,** local anesthesia is not usually required, and sterile surgical gloves are optional as long as care is taken to only touch the hub of the needle (Figure 20.1). The hand holding the needle is placed on the abdomen (for better control of needle advancement), and the needle is thrust through the skin. Then the needle is slowly advanced until it is thought to be in the abdominal cavity. The horse may exhibit a slight pain reaction as the peritoneum is punctured. *Once in the abdomen, the needle hub should not be held because motile intestine moving over a*

stationary needle tip can be lacerated. If the needle hub is observed to move, it is likely that the needle tip is in direct contact with intestine, and the needle should be retracted slightly (Figure 20.2). If peritoneal fluid does not drip from the needle:

   a) the needle can be rotated or advanced further.

   b) additional needles can be inserted cranial or caudal to the original site of centesis.

   c) Aspiration with a syringe is never helpful.

Figure 20.1

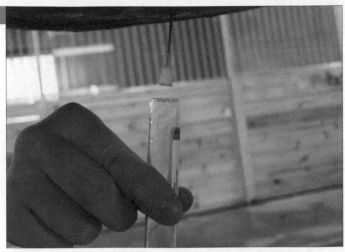

If a hypodermic needle is used for abdominocentesis, local anesthesia is not usually required, and sterile surgical gloves are optional as long as care is taken to only touch the hub of the needle.

Figure 20.2

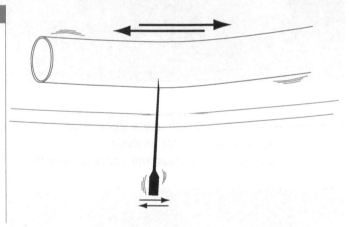

Motile intestine moving over a stationary needle tip can be lacerated. If the needle hub is observed to move, it is likely that the needle tip is in direct contact with intestinal wall.

• **If a teat cannula is used,** local anesthesia is usually required. A stab incision is made through the skin and a portion of the body wall with a #15 blade, and the cannula is advanced until it is thought to be in the abdominal cavity. To avoid contaminating peritoneal fluid with blood from the stab incision, the cannula, before insertion, is passed through a sterile cotton pledget or gauze sponge to absorb dripping blood (Figure 20.3). If peritoneal fluid does not drip from the cannula:

   a) the cannula can be rotated or further advanced.

   b) the hub can be moved to place the cannula tip in a different region of the abdominal cavity.

   c) the cannula can be removed and replaced with a bitch urinary catheter that can be maneuvered into more remote regions of the abdominal cavity in search of fluid (Figure 20.4).

   d) the cannula can be reinserted at another site.

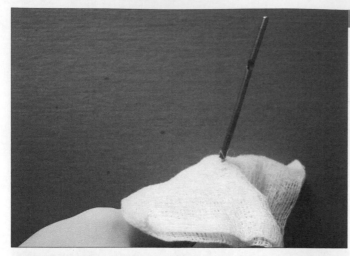

Figure 20.3

To avoid contaminating peritoneal fluid with blood from the stab incision, the cannula, before insertion, is passed through a sterile cotton pledget or gauze sponge to absorb dripping blood.

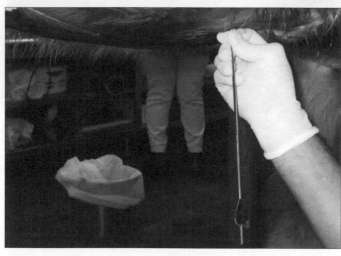

Figure 20.4

A bitch urinary catheter can be maneuvered into more remote regions of the abdominal cavity in search of fluid.

Interpretation

- For evaluation of horses with acute signs of abdominal pain, gross visual examination of peritoneal fluid often is sufficient for analysis.
- Normal peritoneal fluid is **clear and straw-colored** (Figure 20.5).

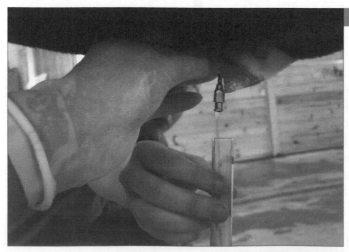

Figure 20.5

Normal peritoneal fluid is clear and straw-colored.

• Fluid with a brownish tint indicates intestinal necrosis, viscal rupture, or enterocentesis (Figure 20.6). Fluid with a **greenish tint** is indicative of viscal rupture or enterocentesis.

• Hemorrhage results in fluid of varying shades of red. If hemorrhage is the result of contamination, the fluid may not be uniformly red as it drips from the cannula or needle. A **reddish or pink tint** remaining in the sample after centrufigation indicates that red blood cells have hemolyzed, and this can occur when intestine has become necrotic. Hemolysis of red blood cells also occurs in chronic conditions, such as neoplasia.

• **Increased turbidity** is usually indicative of increased protein concentration, which occurs in horses with intestinal necrosis or enteritis. Normal peritoneal fluid has a protein concentration less than 1.5 g/dL.

• A horse is considered to have peritonitis when the **nucleated cell count** in the peritoneal fluid is greater than 10,000/uL. The nucleated cell count is normally less than 5,000/uL. Peritonitis can be **septic** or **non-septic.** The presence of **degenerate neutrophils** that may contain phagocitized bacteria indicates that peritonitis is septic.

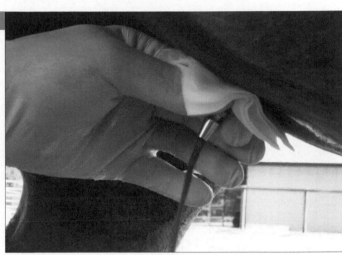

Figure 20.6

Fluid with a brownish tint indicates intestinal necrosis, viscal rupture, or enterocentesis.

Complications

• **Septic peritonitis** can result from enterocentesis. Enterocentesis occurs commonly, especially when the large colon is distended. Enterocentesis is more likely to occur when a hypodermic needle is used for abdominocentesis, but it can also occur when a teat cannula is used. If peritoneal fluid is collected and analyzed several hours after enterocentesis, the nucleated cell count is likely to be high (as high as 500,000 cells/uL), and phagocitized bacteria may be seen. Clinical signs of septic peritonitis subsequent to enterocentesis usually are not apparent (even when enterocentesis occurs when using a teat cannula), except for fever in some horses.

• **Infection at the site of abdominocentesis** may result from enterocentesis, usually in the form of a localized subcutaneous abscess, or cellulitis with multiple abscesses.

• **Intestinal laceration** caused by the tip of a hypodermic needle can occur during abdominocentesis. This complication is more likely to occur in foals, because they are more likely to move during the procedure. A teat cannula, rather than a hypodermic needle, should be used for abdominocentesis of foals.

• **Hemorrhage as the result of splenic puncture** occurs when the spleen lies directly over the site of abdominocentesis. The spleen is more likely to lie over the site of abdominocentesis in horses with displacement of colon over the nephrosplenic ligament or in horses sedated with chloral hydrate. Splenic hemorrhage is usually inconsequential to the health of the horse, but it interferes with cytological analysis of peritoneal fluid.

SUGGESTED READINGS

Ricketts SW. Technique of paracentesis abdominis (peritoneal tap) in the horse. *Equine Veterinary Journal* 15:288-289, 1983.

Nelson AW. Analysis of equine peritoneal fluid. *Veterinary Clinics of North America: Large Animal Practice* 1:267-274, 1979.

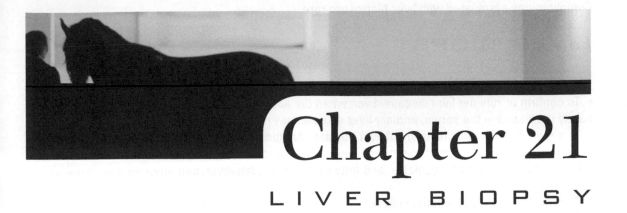

Chapter 21

LIVER BIOPSY

Liver biopsy can be performed safely even when ultrasonographic equipment is not available. Complications associated with liver biopsy are rare.

LIVER BIOPSY

Indications
• To confirm or rule out liver disease. Even when the activity of liver-specific enzymes is significantly increased in the serum, primary liver disease may not be present.
• To supply an etiologic diagnosis of liver disease. An etiologic diagnosis is often not possible because many hepatic diseases produce similar histological changes. Pyrrolizidine alkaloid toxicosis, cholangiohepatitis, neoplasia, and fatty liver disease, however, can often be diagnosed by liver biopsy.
• To provide tissue for bacterial culture
• To determine the prognosis of a horse with liver disease
• To determine the chronicity of disease
• To determine progression or resolution of liver disease (with serial biopsies)

Contraindications
• Horses with advanced cirrhosis may have increased prothrombin and whole-blood clotting times. Coagulopathy is often claimed to be a contraindication for liver biopsy. Significant hemorrhage after liver biopsy is rare, however, even in horses with evidence of a coagulopathy.
• Suspicion of liver abscesses (to avoid bacterial contamination of the thorax and abdomen)
• Concurrent pulmonary disease for which lung biopsy is contraindicated (see section on lung biopsy) because the biopsy needle may pass through lung

Materials
• Sedation is optional, but restraint should be sufficient to prevent movement during the procedure.
• #15 blade and sterile gloves
• 5-10 mL local anesthetic solution
• 12- to 14-gauge biopsy needle (Vim-Silverman, Tru-Cut style, Menghini, or Monopty® are good choices)
• Ultrasonographic equipment for selection of biopsy site (optional) Ultrasonographically guided needle biopsy is useful for diagnosis of focal liver disease.
• 10% formalin and bacterial transport medium

Procedure
• The procedure is performed on the **right side** of the horse
• When ultrasonography is not available to identify the optimum site for liver biopsy, a common site for biopsy is the 14th intercostal space. To find this site, first find the 17th intercostal space (i.e. the last intercostal space) and count forward on a line drawn from the *tuber coxae* to the point of the shoulder (Figure 21.1). When sites cranial to the 14th intercostal space are used, lung is more likely to be penetrated.
• After surgically preparing the biopsy site, the body wall is infiltrated with local anesthetic solution, and the skin is stabbed with a #15 blade near the cranial edge of the neighboring rib (to avoid the intercostal artery located at the caudal edge of each rib).
• The biopsy needle is inserted and directed at a slightly oblique angle (30°) craniad and ventrad, aiming for the opposite elbow (Figure 21.2). If pushed slowly, the biopsy needle can be felt to pass through the diaphragm and enter the liver. The gross appearance of the tissue obtained confirms that a sample of the liver has been collected.

- Tissue is removed from the biopsy needle and placed in formalin, and if bacterial cholangiohepatitis is suspected, another sample of tissue is collected and placed in a bacterial transport medium.
- The stab incision can be closed with a suture or allowed to heal by second intention.

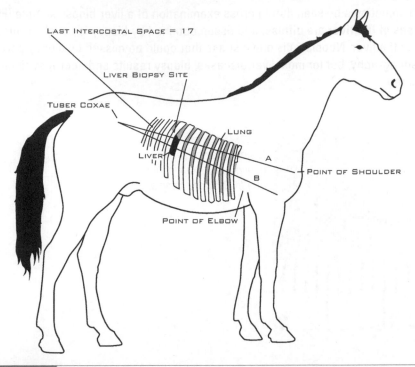

Figure 21.1 *A common site for blind liver biopsy is the 14th intercostal space near a line drawn from the tuber coxae to the point of the shoulder.*

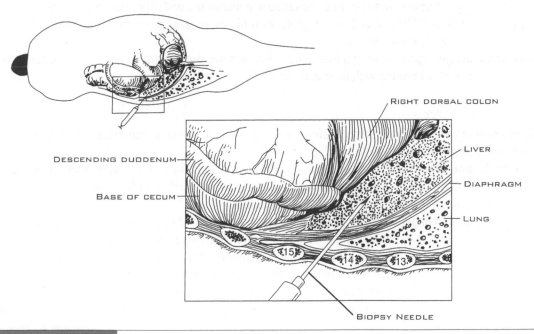

Figure 21.2 *The biopsy needle is inserted and directed at a slightly oblique angle (30°) craniad and ventrad aiming for the opposite elbow.*

Interpretation

A histopathologist should interpret the biopsy, but a brief histological description of some liver diseases is presented.

• Lesions can sometimes be seen during gross examination of a liver biopsy sample (Figure 21.3).

• **Most diseases of the liver are diffuse,** and tissue obtained by biopsy is usually representative of the condition of the liver. Neoplasia is one disease that could be missed by biopsy performed without ultrasonography, but for most liver diseases, biopsy results and necropsy findings are closely correlated.

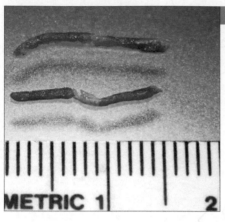

Figure 21.3

Lesions may be seen during gross examination of a liver biopsy sample.

• Pyrrolizidine alkaloid poisoning, one of the most common causes of liver disease in the horse, causes typical changes in the liver: hepatomegalocytosis, proliferation of bile ducts, and periportal fibrosis.

• The bile ducts of horses with cholangiohepatitis are distended with purulent debris, and surrounding tissue is infiltrated with neutrophils. Aerobic or anaerobic bacteria can often be cultured from the biopsy specimens.

• Histopathological examination of a liver biopsy has greater prognostic value than other tests for determining survival of horses with liver disease.

Complications

• **Complications are rare** if contraindications are not ignored. Owners should be warned, however, of potential complications.

• **Hepatic hemorrhage.** For horses with clinicopathological evidence of a coagulopathy, transfusion of two liters of blood may prevent hemmorhage. Significant hemorrhage after liver biopsy is rare, however, even in horses with evidence of a coagulopathy.

• **Pulmonary hemorrhage.** Because the biopsy needle may pass through lung, severe pulmonary hemorrhage may occur, especially if the horse has recurrent airway obstruction.

• **Biopsy of other organs.** When this occurs, most commonly it is the lung that is biopsied. Lung tissue is easily identified by gross examination. Intestinal contents are occasionally found in the biopsy needle. If intestinal contents are retrieved, the biopsy is repeated at another site using another sterile biopsy instrument, and as a precaution, broad-spectrum antimicrobial drugs can be administered for several days.

SUGGESTED READINGS

Pearson EG, Craig AM. The diagnosis of liver disease in equine and food animals. Modern Veterinary Practice 61: 233-237, 1980.

Pearson EG. Liver disease in the mature horse. Equine Veterinary Education 11:87-96, 1999.

Durham AE, Smith KC, Newton JR, Hillyer MH, Hillyer LL, Smith MR, Marr CM. Development and application of a scoring system for prognostic evaluation of equine liver biopsies. Equine Veterinary Journal 35:534-540, 2003.

Chapter 22

RECTAL MUCOSAL

BIOPSY

Rectal mucosa is easily biopsied with little risk to the horse.

RECTAL MUCOSAL BIOPSY

Indications
• Acute or chronic diarrhea. Concurrent culture of rectal mucosa and feces increases the likeli-hood of isolating *Salmonella spp.* compared to fecal culture alone. Diarrhea of some horses is associated with the infiltration of mucosa and submucosa with populations of inflammatory (i.e., infiltrative bowel disease) or neoplastic cells, and for some of these horses, lesions can be found, and diagnosis made, by histological examination of rectal mucosa.
• Weight-loss attributed to intestinal disease. Rectal biopsy may aid in the diagnosis of intestinal lymphosarcoma and some types of idiopathic infiltrative bowel disease. For some horses with gran-ulomatous enteritis or multisystemic, eosinophilic, epitheliotropic disease, *antemortem* diagnosis is made by histological examination of rectal mucosa. Lymphocytic-plasmacytic enterocolitis and eosinophilic enterocolitis are unlikely to be diagnosed by histological examination of rectal mucosa.

Contraindications
• The procedure can be dangerous for the horse or the clinician taking the sample, if the horse is fractious and not easily controlled.
• **Tenesmus** The procedure can be dangerous for horses with acute diarrhea, because an arm in the rectum of these horses can cause them to strain, which can result in rectal injury. (Caudal epidural anesthesia may prevent straining during rectal biopsy of horses with acute diarrhea.)

Materials
• An alligator-type biopsy forceps (such as a mare endometrial biopsy forceps)
• A small gauge, hypodermic needle to remove the specimen from the forceps
• Lubrication and an obstetrical sleeve
• 10% formalin and a bacterial transport medium. Bouin's solution is a poor choice for a fixative for rectal mucosa, because it makes eosinophils less conspicuous.

Procedure
• Restraint is the same as for safe palpation of the abdomen *per rectum.*
• The rectum is cleared of feces. Proctoscopic examination, using a tube vaginal speculum or a colonoscope, may aid in identifying areas of disease for biopsy.
• The closed jaws of the biopsy forceps are protected by a lubricated hand and carried into the rectum to elbow depth (Figure 22.1).

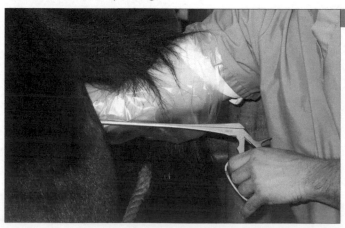

Figure 22.1
The closed jaws of the biopsy forceps are protected by a lubricated hand and carried into the rectum to elbow depth.

• The jaws of the forceps are opened, and rectal mucosa from the 10 or 2 o'clock region of the rectum is grasped between the thumb and index finger and pulled into the jaws of the biopsy forceps (Figure 22.2). The dorsal aspect of the rectum should not be biopsied to avoid trauma to the rectal vasculature.

• Mucosa can be placed directly in fixative, but by orienting the tissue on filter paper, sections can be taken at right angles to the surface for better histological evaluation.

• Mucosa for bacteriologic culture is placed in an enrichment medium or physiologic saline solution and then chilled for transport.

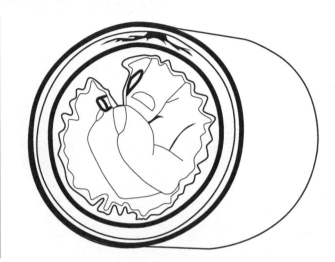

Figure 22.2

The jaws of the forceps are opened, and rectal mucosa from the 10 or 2 o'clock region of the rectum is grasped between the thumb and index finger and pulled into the jaws of the biopsy forceps.

Interpretation

• *Salmonella spp.* is often cultured from rectal mucosa of horses with salmonellosis, even when fecal cultures are negative for the organism.

• Rectal biopsy is often helpful for diagnosis of infiltrative bowel disease. A histopathologist interprets the biopsy, but a brief histological description of some intestinal diseases is presented.

» Sheets of macrophages or epitheliod cells and circumscribed granulomas in the mucosa or submucosa are seen during histological examination of rectal mucosa of horses with *granulomatous enteritis.*

» Lymphoid and plasma cells can be found in rectal tissue of horses with various intestinal diseases. Finding a lymphocytic-proctitis during histological examination of rectal tissue, particularly if lymphocytic infiltration is mild, may not justify a diagnosis of *lymphocytic-plasmacytic enteritis.*

» *Eosinophilic enterocolitis* is unlikely to be diagnosed based on results of a rectal biopsy, because eosinophilic infiltrates can be found in the rectal mucosa of normal horses. The presence of eosinophilic granulomas associated with vasculitis and fibrinoid necrosis of intramural vessels in rectal tissue is considered diagnostic of *multisystemic, eosinophilic, epitheliotropic disease.*

Complications

• **Complications are very unlikely.** *Post mortem* examination of horses that have had their rectal mucosa biopsied indicates that the biopsy site is healed within 3 days and is difficult or impossible to find after 5 days.

• Trauma from recent palpations *per rectum* can cause histological changes in the mucosa. Biopsies intended for histological examination should, therefore, be taken from the dorsolateral aspect of the rectum and before extensive palpation is performed.

SUGGESTED READINGS

Palmer JE, Whitlock RH, Benson CE, *et. al.* Comparison of rectal mucosal cultures and fecal cultures in detecting Salmonella infection in horses and cattle. *American Journal of Veterinary Research* 46:697-698, 1985.

Lindberg R, Nygren A, Persson SGB. Rectal biopsy diagnosis in horses with clinical signs of intestinal disorders: A retrospective study of 116 cases. *Equine Veterinary Journal* 28:275-284, 1996.

Chapter 23

MUSCLE BIOPSY

Within recent years different diseases associated with rhabdomyolysis and muscle wasting in the horse have been identified. Accurate diagnosis of muscle disease is important because prognosis and long-term management of these diseases often differ. Because these diseases have similar clinical and clinicopathological signs, an accurate diagnosis often depends on histopathological examination of muscle.

MUSCLE BIOPSY

• Muscle biopsy samples can be collected using incisional (open) or needle biopsy techniques. Needle biopsy of muscle is simple, rapidly performed, and usually, the horse can continue training. Using a needle to obtain a sample of muscle requires some practice and skill and the specialized needle used for muscle biopsy, while reusable, is expensive to purchase. Incisional (open) biopsy is more likely to provide a diagnostic sample of muscle than is needle biopsy, but this method of biopsy requires several days of confinement and restricted exercise and is more often associated with minor complications. Interpretation of a muscle biopsy may be enhanced if both apparently normal and abnormal muscle tissue is submitted for evaluation. **Before a muscle biopsy is taken, laboratory personnel should be consulted for instructions concerning preparation of tissue for shipment.**

Indications
• To aid in diagnosis of muscular or neuromuscular diseases such as equine glycogen storage disorders (polysaccharide storage myopathy and glycogen branching enzyme deficiency), equine motor neuron disease, recurrent exertional rhabdomyolysis, white muscle disease, inflammatory or immune-mediated myositis, or myositis caused by some *Sarcocystis sp.*
• To aid in evaluating the prognosis of horses with muscle disease by determining the degree of muscle cell degeneration and the amount of muscle fiber replacement with fibrous tissue
• For research in equine exercise physiology

Materials
• A sedative
• Stocks are useful.
• Local anesthetic solution
• A #10 and a #22 scalpel blade
• Sterile surgical gloves
For incisional biopsy:
» Absorbable and nonabsorbable suture material or skin staples of appropriate size
» Tongue depressor or cardboard, and several fine-gauge needles, or a commercially available, muscle biopsy clamp (Price Muscle Biopsy Clamp or Rayport Muscle Biopsy Clamp, V. Mueller, Allegiance Healthcare Corporation, McGaw Park, IL 60085 USA) (Figure 23.1) (optional)
For needle biopsy:
» A 5 mm or larger muscle biopsy needle (Carl Mortensen, Spanagervej 25, 4632 Bjaevrskov, Denmark; Popper & Sons, Inc. 300 Denton Ave., New Hyde Park, NY 11040 USA) (Figures 1.9, 23.2)
» An 8- or 9-mm skin biopsy punch can be used to biopsy superficial regions of muscle (i.e., the *sacrocaudalis dorsalis medialis* **muscle** for diagnosis of equine motor neuron disease) (Figure 23.3)
• Sterile gauze sponge
• 10% buffered formalin
• Ice packs for shipment (optional)
• Dry ice for shipment (optional)

Figure 23.1

Commercially available, stainless steel and plastic, disposable, muscle biopsy clamps are shown.

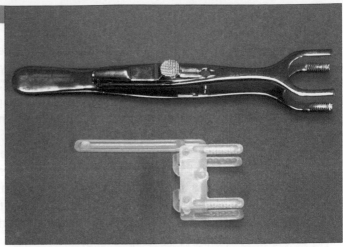

Figure 23.2

Two types of commercially available, muscle biopsy instruments are shown.

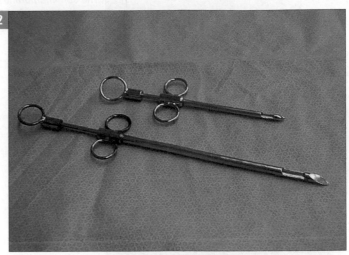

Figure 23.3

An 8- or 9-mm skin biopsy punch can be used to biopsy superficial regions of muscle (i.e., the sacrocaudalis dorsalis medialis muscle for diagnosis of equine motor neuron disease).

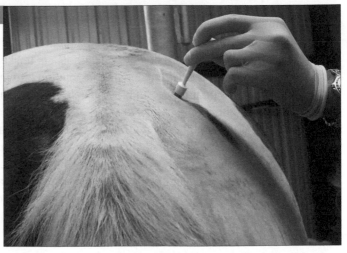

Procedure

• The horse is sedated.

• The site of biopsy is chosen according to the disease suspected. Biopsy of the **semimembranosus muscle** is recommended if equine polysaccharide storage myopathy is suspected. This muscle is biopsied approximately 10 cm below the *tuber ischii* (Figure 23.4). The **sacrocaudalis dorsalis medialis muscle** is biopsied if equine motor neuron disease is suspected, and histological evaluation of muscle from both of these sites may clarify a diagnosis, when clinical and clinicopathologic signs correlate with either of these diseases. When equine polysaccharide storage myopathy is suspected as the cause of back pain, the **longissimus lumborum muscle** is biopsied. For horses suspected of having recurrent exertional myopathy, the **middle gluteal muscle** is commonly biopsied. The **longissimus lumborum muscle** is biopsied behind the saddle region 5 to 7 cm off the midline at a depth of 3 to 4 cm. The **middle gluteal muscle** is biopsied, at a depth of 6 cm, 18 cm from the *tuber coxae* on a line connecting the dorsum of the *tuber coxae* to the tail head (Figure 23.5).

• The biopsy site is prepared for aseptic surgery.

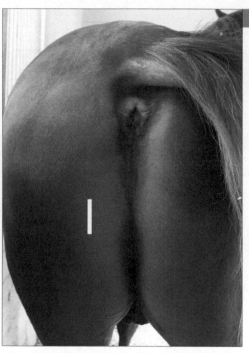

Figure 23.4

The semimembranosus muscle is biopsied approximately 10 cm below the tuber ischii.

• **For incisional (open) biopsy:**

» Local anesthetic solution is administered subcutaneously at the site of biopsy in an inverted U-pattern, or in a line; caudal epidural anesthesia is unlikely to provide adequate analgesia of the biopsy site. Avoid injecting local anesthetic solution into muscle.

» A 5-cm skin incision is made, and the muscle fascia is incised to expose **muscle fibers that run parallel with the incision.**

» Two parallel incisions, 1- cm apart and 3- to 5- cm long are made in the muscle.

» A curved scissors or a hemostat is used to bluntly undermine muscle between the two incisions before ends of the specimen are cut. The size of the muscle specimen can be varied with the length of the incision and the depth of blunt dissection. Procuring a 3- to 5- cm strip of muscle is recommended for diagnosis of equine polysaccharide storage myopathy or equine motor neuron disease.

» A commercially available muscle biopsy clamp, which minimizes contraction artifact, can be used to secure the muscle before it is cut. Or muscle is attached to the tongue depressor or cardboard

Figure 23.5A & B

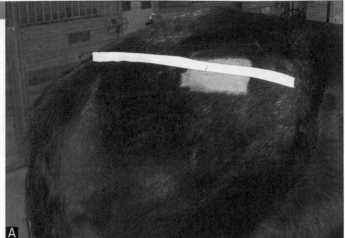

(A) and *(B)* The middle gluteal muscle is biopsied, at a depth of 6 cm, 18 cm from the tuber coxae on a line connecting the tuber coxae to the tail head.

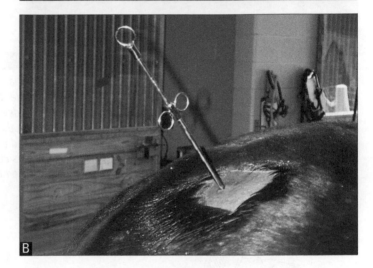

with needles placed through each end of undermined muscle (Figure 23.6). Then the strip of muscle is cut at each end. *If a 1- x 1- x 5- cm or larger sample of muscle is obtained, securing the muscle is not necessary. Large samples can be accurately interpreted, despite contraction artifacts.*

» Muscle fascia is closed using absorbable suture, and the subcutis is closed with absorbable suture. These two tissue layers are closed using a simple continuous pattern. Skin is closed with nonabsorbable suture in a simple interrupted or vertical mattress pattern or with skin staples.

» A gauze stent can be sutured over the wound.

- **For needle biopsy:**

  » Skin at the site of biopsy is anesthetized with a subcutaneous bleb of local anesthetic solution. Avoid injecting local anesthetic solution into muscle.

  » A stab incision, through skin and muscle fascia, is made with a scalpel blade.
  The biopsy needle is inserted into muscle. The needle is forced sideways to force tissue into the cutting cylinder, and a section of muscle is cut using the inner core of the needle (Figure 23.7).

  » Skin can be closed or left unsutured.

- The specimen is placed in 10% buffered formalin. Or, specimens can be wrapped in gauze *lightly* moistened with physiologic saline solution for shipment in a watertight container surrounded by ice packs. Or samples can be frozen immediately in isopentane cooled in liquid nitrogen and placed in plastic bags for shipment on dry ice.

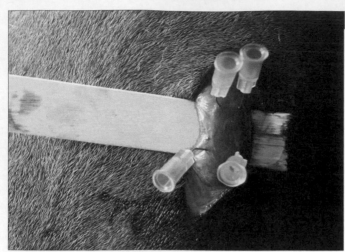

Figure 23.6

If a commercially available, muscle biopsy clamp, which minimizes contraction artifact, is not available, muscle can be attached to a tongue depressor or cardboard by placing needles through each end of undermined muscle, before severing the muscle.

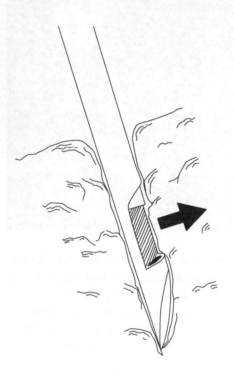

Figure 23.7

The biopsy needle is inserted into muscle, the needle is forced sideways to force tissue into the cutting cylinder, and a section of muscle is cut using the inner core of the needle.

Complications

Complications of incisional biopsy include:

• **Seroma or hematoma** at the biopsy site. This complication can be ignored, or the hematoma or seroma can be drained using a needle and syringe or several sutures can be removed to allow continuous drainage.

• The owner should be warned that **wound dehiscence** is a common complication with incisional biopsy of the *semimembranosus* or *semitendinosus* muscle. To lessen the likelihood of dehiscence, the horse should be confined to a stall for five to seven days after biopsy and not heavily exercised for two weeks. The owner can be reassured that an open wound in this area will heal by second intention within several weeks.

Complications of needle biopsy include:

- Localized swelling that resolves in several days
- Sampling error. Focal lesions might be missed because of the small size of the biopsy specimen (multiple biopsies might prevent this problem).
- Small samples are difficult to orient properly for histological examination.

Interpretation

A pathologist familiar with the histological appearance of equine myopathies should evaluate muscle biopsies, but brief histological descriptions of some muscle diseases are presented.

- Muscle fibers of horses with **equine polysaccharide storage myopathy** contain *complex polysaccharide* that stains bright pink/purple with periodic acid-Schiff (PAS) stain and grey-blue with hematoxylin and eosin (H&E) stain. Complex polysaccharide resists digestion with amylase and diagnosis is confirmed by subjecting specimens to amylase digestion before staining. Most researchers believe that amylase-resistant complex polysaccharide *must* be seen before equine polysaccharide storage myopathy can be diagnosed, but some believe that finding excessive glycogen in the muscle, along with non-specific histological signs of muscle disease, is sufficient for diagnosis.
- Skeletal muscle of foals affected with **glycogen branching enzyme deficiency** contains abnormal PAS positive globular or crystalline intracellular inclusions.
- Typically, affected muscle fibers at different stages of degeneration and regeneration are seen in horses with **recurrent exertional rhabdomyolysis.** Histopathological lesions are nonspecific and may include focal necrosis, vacuolated and fragmented fibers, fibers infiltrated with macrophages, and regenerative fibers with central nuclei, fatty infiltration and fibrosis. Horses with recurrent exertional rhabdomyolysis may also have muscle fibers that have increased PAS staining for glycogen, but this glycogen does not resist digestion with amylase.
- Denervation atrophy resulting in clusters of atrophied muscle fibers and adjacent hypertrophied fibers are typical findings in horses with **equine motor neuron disease,** equine protozoal myelitis, and nerve trauma. Demyelination of intramuscular nerves may be observed (nerves are not always present in sections) when muscle is stained with Masson's trichrome, which stains myelin red.

SUGGESTED READINGS

Andrews FM, Reed SM, Johnson GC. Muscle biopsy in the horse: Its indications, techniques, and complications. *Veterinary Medicine* 88:357-365,1993.

Quiroz-Rothe E, Novales M, Aguilera-Tejero E, Rivero LL. Polysaccharide storage myopathy in the M. longissimus lumborum of showjumpers and dressage horses with back pain. *Equine Veterinary Journal* 34:171-176, 2002.

Valberg SJ, MacLeay JM, Mickelson JR. Exertional rhabdomyolysis and polysaccharide storage myopathy in horses. *Compendium of Continuing Education for the Practicing Veterinarian* 19:1077-1085, 1997.

Valberg SJ. Spinal muscle pathology. *Veterinary Clinics of North America: Equine Practice* 15:87-95,1999.

Valentine BA, Divers TJ, Murphy DJ, Todhunter PG. Muscle biopsy diagnosis of equine motor neuron disease and equine polysaccharide storage myopathy. *Equine Veterinary Education* 10:42-50, 1998.

Chapter 24

SYNOVIOCENTESIS

There may be more than one reported method to access a joint or tendon sheath. In this chapter, only one method is presented (the one preferred by the authors). Also there is a trend among practitioners to use smaller gauge needles (than recommended in this chapter) for centesis of some joints. This is personal preference and should be considered. Use of a smaller gauge needle may facilitate synoviocentesis of some fractious horses, and may cause less synovial hemorrhage. These needles are more likely to break, however, if the horse moves during synoviocentesis.

SYNOVIOCENTESIS

Indications
- To collect synovial fluid for cytological analysis or bacteriological culture
- To administer local anesthetic solution as part of a lameness examination or to administer medication such as a corticosteroid or sodium hyaluronate
- To administer a polyionic fluid or radiocontrast material to check for communication of a joint or tendon sheath with a nearby wound

Materials
- Hair clippers are optional. Traditionally, the site of centesis is clipped prior to needle puncture, but a recent study and experience of some practitioners indicate that clipping is not necessary, if the area is properly scrubbed. Some owners may be more satisfied if the hair is left unclipped.
- An antiseptic soap, such as povidine-iodine or chlorhexadine
- 70% isopropyl alcohol
- Sterile, surgical gloves
- At least two sterile, disposable needles A 20-ga (0.90 mm) needle is commonly used to administer drugs. The needle used to draw medication from a bottle should not be used for joint injection. A new needle should be used for each injection.
- To lessen the likelihood of sepsis, a **new, unused bottle** of drug should be used for joint injection.
- A lip twitch
- A sedative (best avoided if synoivocentesis is part of a lameness examination) If application of a lip twitch or lip chain does not provide sufficient restraint for synoviocentesis as part of a lameness examination, the horse can be sedated with xylazine HCL or detomidine often without interfering significantly with assessment of gait. The degree to which sedation may interfere with assessment of gait, however, may depend upon the severity of lameness and the skill of the clinician performing the lameness examination.
- **Fluid for cytological examination** is collected in EDTA tubes. Fluid for bacterial culture can be collected in a capped, air-free syringe for immediate delivery to the laboratory, or if a delay in submission is anticipated, synovial fluid can be collected into Port-A-Cul tubes or vials.
- **For intrasynovial analgesia,** *mepivacaine* is the local anesthetic solution most commonly administered because it is relatively non-irritating to tissues. The analgesic effect of mepivacaine lasts about 2 hours. *Lidocaine* is irritating to tissue and produces analgesia for only 30 to 40 minutes.

Procedure
- The site of needle placement is scrubbed for at least 5 minutes and then rinsed with alcohol.
- For some joints, multiple sites for needle placement have been described. In this text, the examples illustrated are the sites preferred by the authors.
- Not all horses respond in the same way to different methods of restraint, but for most horses, application of a lip twitch provides adequate restraint. The twitch works best when applied immediately

prior to needle placement. When a joint is injected with the horse's limb on the ground, the contralateral limb can be lifted off the ground to enhance the safety of the procedure for the clinician. Clinicians should be aware, however, that some horses might buckle in the knee of the weight-bearing limb and fall when the needle is introduced.

• Synovial fluid is usually more easily collected as it drips from the needle than by aspiration with a syringe. An alternative technique to aspirate synovial fluid involves inserting one end of a blood collection needle into the joint, inserting the other end of the needle into a blood collection tube, and allowing the tube to fill (Figure 24.1).

• If a sufficient quantity of synovial fluid cannot be collected for bacterial culture, aspirating the joint after infusing it with physiological saline solution usually allows enough fluid to be collected for culture.

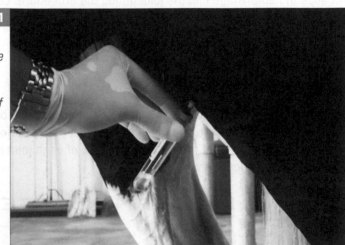

Figure 24.1

Synovial fluid can be collected by inserting one end of a blood collection needle into the joint, inserting the other end of the needle into a blood collection tube and allowing the tube to fill.

Interpretation

• Normal synovial fluid is pale yellow and clear. The amount of fluid collected varies, but more fluid can usually be obtained from diseased joints.

• Red blood cells are not a normal constituent of synovial fluid, but blood frequently contaminates synovial fluid during synoviocentesis. Streaks of blood within the sample usually indicate contamination at the time of collection. Dark yellow to amber samples may indicate chronic traumatic arthritis. Marked increase in the number of red blood cells may also indicate sepsis.

• Clotting of the sample indicates severe inflammation of the joint or tendon sheath. Synovial fluid from healthy tendon sheaths and joints or joints affected by degenerative disease does not clot.

• Protein concentration is normally < 2.0 g/dL.

• Cell count is normally less than 600 nucleated cells/uL, most of which are small lymphocytes and monocytes.

• Indications of sepsis are:
   » a predominance of segmented neutrophils (often > than 30,000 cells/µL)
   » degenerate neutrophils (In contrast to morphology of neutrophils found in other infected body fluids, however, neutrophils in septic synovial fluid often appear healthy and have little or no degenerative changes.)
   » fluid that clots
   » a turbulent fluid
   » a protein concentration > 4 gm/dL
   » culture of bacterial colonies. At least one-fourth of samples of septic synovial fluid yield no bacterial growth.

Complications

• *Iatrogenic sepsis* is an unlikely complication of synoviocentesis, as long as the procedure is performed using sterile technique. Some clinicians routinely administer an antibiotic during synoviocentesis, but we consider this practice usually to be unnecessary, even when an immunosupressive drug, such as a corticosteroid is administered intra-synovially. However, because infection occasionally occurs after intra-synovial administration of polysulphated glycosaminoglycan, we suggest that 150 to 200 mg of amikacin be administered along with this drug.

• *Blood contamination* of a sample of synovial fluid is common, because the synovial membrane is very vascular.

• Hemarthrosis. Some horses display signs of acute pain following arthrocentesis, possibly because of hemorrhage into the joint during the procedure. Lameness caused by hemarthrosis usually resolves within 24 hours.

ARTHROCENTESIS

Techniques

For some joints, multiple techniques for arthrocentesis have been described. In this section, we describe the techniques that we believe are most easily performed. The optimal amount of local anesthetic agent required for optimal analgesia of each joint has not been established, and volumes stated are only suggestions.

DISTAL INTERPHALANGEAL (COFFIN) JOINT

Lateral, palmar and dorsal approaches for arthrocentesis have been described for this joint. Using the lateral or palmar approach, however, the navicular bursa or the digital flexor tendon sheath can occasionally be penetrated. We prefer a dorsal approach where the needle enters the dorsal pouch of the distal interphalangeal (DIP) joint. *The clinician should be aware that the following technique might be more dangerous to perform than techniques in which the foot can be held off the ground.*

Materials

• 20- ga, 1 inch (0.90 x 25mm) sterile, disposable needles
• 5 to 6mL local anesthetic solution if intra-articular analgesia is required
• Sterile surgical gloves
• Lip twitch

Technique

• Arthrocentesis is performed with the limb bearing weight.
• For some horses, the procedure may be more safely performed by lifting the contralateral limb; however some horses, with the contralateral limb held, may fall to their knees when the needle is inserted. *Application of a lip twitch is indicated for this procedure.*
• The needle is inserted through the coronary band *parallel or* slightly oblique to the bearing surface at the dorsal midline (Figure 24.2). Because the dorsal pouch of the DIP joint extends proximally for several centimeters, the joint is fairly easily accessed using the dorsal parallel approach (Figure 24.3). (Although some anatomical drawings of the foot show the extensor process of the distal phalanx to extend above the coronary band, the extensor process lies below the coronary band.) Firm digital pressure for several seconds at this site before the needle is inserted may

decrease pain and reaction from the horse. Some horses react violently to insertion of the needle by thrusting the limb upwards. To safely perform the procedure, the clinician and person holding the horse should anticipate this reaction and position themselves accordingly.

• Some clinicians, using the dorsal approach, insert the needle through a site on the midline one cm dorsal to coronary band, *perpendicular* to the bearing surface. This technique is more difficult to perform than the one just described.

• Fluid may drip from the needle, but correct placement of the needle is also indicated by easy injection of drug; the syringe may refill when pressure is removed from the plunger after injection.

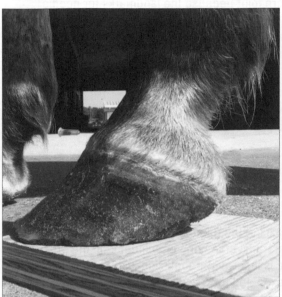
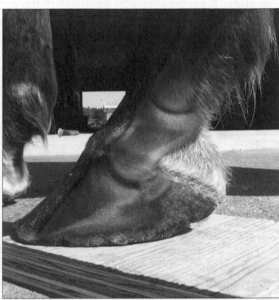

Figure 24.2   To place a needle into the coffin joint, the needle is inserted through the coronary band at the dorsal midline, parallel to the bearing surface.

Figure 24.3

Because the dorsal pouch of the DIP joint extends proximally for several centimeters, the joint is easily accessed using the dorsal parallel approach. Six mL of radiocontrast solution were administered into this DIP joint.

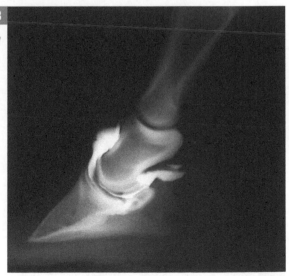

Interpretation

• Analgesia of the DIP joint, using 5 or 6 mL of local anesthetic solution, also causes analgesia of the **navicular apparatus,** the **toe region of the sole,** and, probably, a **portion of the third phalanx.**

Administration of a larger volume of local anesthetic solution (i.e., 10mL) causes analgesia of the heel region of the sole.

• The gait should be evaluated 10 minutes after analgesia of the DIP joint. If evaluation of gait is delayed, diffusion of local anesthetic solution may result in desensitization of the heel region of the sole.

PROXIMAL INTERPHALANGEAL (PASTERN) JOINT

We prefer the palmar/plantar approach to the pastern joint because the landmarks for needle placement are obvious, because synovial fluid is often obtained to verify proper needle placement, and because the foot is held, making the procedure safer than a dorsal approach where the needle is inserted with the limb bearing weight.

Materials
• 20- ga, 1 inch (0.90 x 25 mm) sterile, disposable needles
• 4mL local anesthetic solution if intra-articular analgesia is required
• Sterile surgical gloves
• Lip twitch

Technique
• The procedure is performed with the limb held.
• The needle is inserted perpendicular to the long axis of the pastern, close to the palmar border of the first phalanx, just proximal to the easily palpable transverse bony prominence on the proximopalmar aspect of the middle phalanx. The needle is inserted through skin with the joints of the lower limb in extension and then these joints are flexed and the needle is advanced into the proximal interphalangeal (PIP) joint (Figure 24.4). Because the palmar pouch of the (PIP) joint extends proximally for several centimeters the joint is fairly easily accessed using the palmar/plantar approach (Figure 24.5).
• Synovial fluid may drip from the needle.

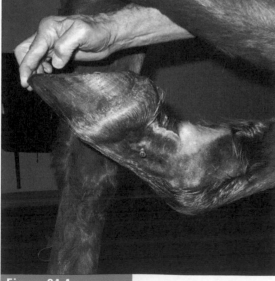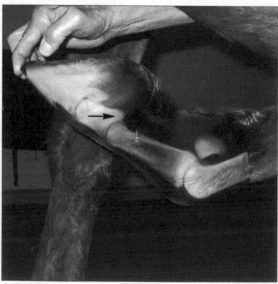

Figure 24.4   *For arthrocentesis of the proximal interphalangeal joint, a needle is inserted perpendicular to the long axis of the pastern, close to the caudal border of the first phalanx, just proximal to the transverse bony prominence on the proximopalmar aspect of the middle phalanx (arrow).*

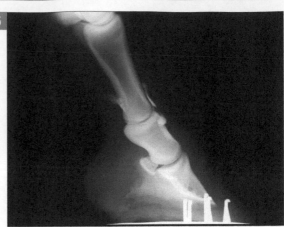

Figure 24.5

Because the palmar pouch of the PIP joint extends proximally for several centimeters this joint is fairly easily accessed using the palmar/plantar approach. Four mL of radiocontrast solution were administered into this PIP joint.

METACARPOPHALANGEAL (FETLOCK) JOINT

Arthrocentesis of the fetlock joint performed using a lateropalmar approach in which the needle is inserted through the lateral collateral sesamoidian ligament is less likely to cause hemarthosis and subcutaneous inflammation than arthrocentsis through the proximal palmar pouch. This technique can be performed solo, but having the limb held in a flexed position by an assistant is helpful.

Materials
- 20-ga, 1.5 inch (0.90 x 38 mm) sterile, disposable needle
- 5 to 10mL local anesthetic solution if intra-articular analgesia is required
- Sterile surgical gloves
- Lip twitch

Technique
- The procedure is best performed from the lateral side with an assistant flexing the joint.
- A needle is inserted through the lateral collateral sesamoidian ligament between the articular surfaces of the distal metacarpus/tarsus and the lateral proximal sesamoid bone (Figure 24.6). The ligament is the distal border of a depression formed, when the fetlock is flexed, by the palmar surface of the third metacarpus/metatarsus and the dorsal surface of the lateral, proximal sesamoid bone.
- Synovial fluid is usually observed to drip from the needle.

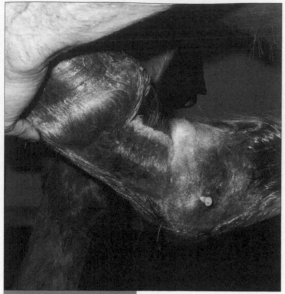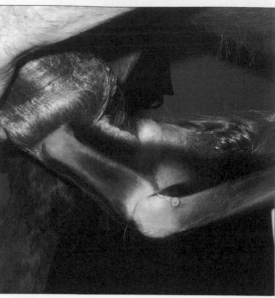

Figure 24.6 *For arthrocentesis of the metacarpo(metatarso)phalangeal joint, a needle is inserted through the lateral collateral sesamoidian ligament. The ligament is the distal border of a depression formed, when the fetlock is flexed, by the palmar surface of the third metacarpus/metatarsus and the dorsal surface of the lateral, proximal sesamoid bone.*

CARPAL JOINTS

The carpus consists of 3 principal joints: radiocarpal (antebrachiocarpal), intercarpal (middle carpal or midcarpal), and carpometacarpal. The carpometacarpal joint communicates with the intercarpal joint so accessing the small carpometacarpal joint directly is unnecessary. The radiocarpal and intercarpal joints can be accessed from either a dorsal or a palmarolateral approach. The palmaro-lateral approach is more difficult but can be performed with the limb bearing weight.

INTERCARPAL (MIDDLE OR MIDCARPAL) JOINT

Materials
- 20-ga, 1.0 inch (0.90 x 25 mm) sterile, disposable needles
- 10mL local anesthetic solution if intra-articular analgesia is required
- Sterile surgical gloves
- Lip twitch

Technique
- The procedure is performed with the carpus flexed. Some clinicians prefer an assistant to hold the limb, but one person can, usually without difficulty, lift the limb and insert a needle while maintaining sterility.
- The joint can be accessed medial or lateral to the tendon of the extensor *carpi radialis* muscle, but for ease, the lateral side is usually chosen. The joint, when flexed, is easily identified by a depression on either side of the tendon (Figure 24.7).

- The needle should be inserted no further than 0.5 inch (12.6 mm) and slightly proximad to avoid damaging articular cartilage.
- Care should be taken to insert the needle at the center of the depression to avoid the tendon sheaths of the extensor *carpi radialis* and common digital extensor muscles.

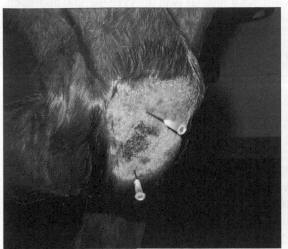 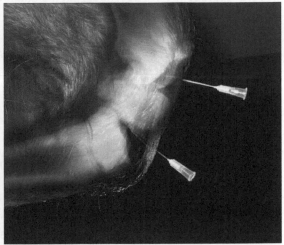

Figure 24.7 *For arthrocentesis of the radiocarpal or intercarpal joint, a needle is inserted medial or lateral to the tendon of the extensor carpi radialis muscle. The joints, when flexed, are easily identified as depressions on either side of the tendon. The higher needle has been placed in the radiocarpal joint and the lower needle has been placed in the intercarpal joint.*

RADIOCARPAL CARPAL (ANTEBRACHIOCARPAL) JOINT

Materials
- 20- ga, 1.0 inch (0.90 x 25 mm) sterile, disposable needles
- 10mL local anesthetic solution if intra-articular analgesia is required
- Sterile surgical gloves
- Lip twitch

Technique
- The procedure is performed with the carpus flexed. Some clinicians prefer an assistant to hold the limb, but one person can usually, without difficulty, lift the limb and insert a needle in a sterile manner.
- The joint can be accessed medial or lateral to the tendon of the extensor *carpi radialis* muscle. The joint, when flexed, is easily identified as a depression on either side of the tendon (Figure 24.7). Because the depression on the lateral side is smaller and, thus, slightly less accessible, the medial side is sometimes chosen for arthrocentesis.
- Care should be taken to avoid penetrating the tendon sheaths of the extensor *carpi radialis* and common digital extensor muscles.

HUMORORADIAL, HUMOROULNAR, AND RADIOULNAR (ELBOW) JOINT(S)

Because disease of the elbow joint is uncommon, arthrocentesis of this joint is seldom performed. Several approaches are described, but the authors are more familiar with the craniolateral approach.

Materials

- 20- ga, 1.5 inch (0.90 x 38 mm) sterile, disposable needles
- 10 to 15mL local anesthetic solution if intra-articular analgesia is required
- Sterile surgical gloves
- Lip twitch

Technique

- The procedure is performed with the limb bearing weight.
- Landmarks for injection are the lateral humeral epicondyle, the lateral tuberosity of the radius, and the lateral collateral ligament connecting these structures.
- The needle is inserted caudomedially at the cranial edge of the lateral, collateral ligament, two-thirds of the distance from the humeral epicondyle to the lateral tuberosity of the radius (Figure 24.8). *Because periarticular administration of local anesthetic agent near the elbow joint can anesthetize motor nerves, some clinicians prefer to inject a relatively short-acting, local anesthetic solution (e.g., lidocaine), to avoid prolonged paralysis of the limb, if this complication occurs. Alternatively, saline can be injected and then aspirated to determine if the needle is placed correctly, before local anesthetic solution is administered.*

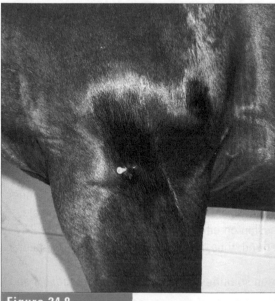 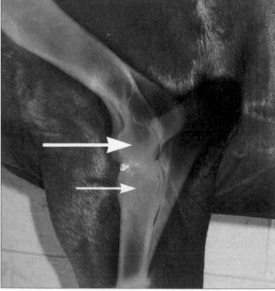

Figure 24.8 *For arthrocentesis of the radiohumeral joint, a needle is inserted craniomedially at the caudal edge (or caudomedially at the cranial edge) of the lateral, collateral ligament, two-thirds of the distance from the humeral epicondyle (upper arrow) to the lateral tuberosity of the radius (lower arrow).*

SCAPULOHUMERAL (SHOULDER) JOINT

Because, for some horses, the shoulder joint communicates with the bicipital bursa, intra-articular administration of local anesthetic solution might anesthetize both structures.

Materials
- 18- or 20-ga, 3.5-inch (1.2- or 0.9- x 8.89-cm) sterile, disposable spinal needle
- 20 to 30mL local anesthetic solution if intra-articular analgesia is required
- Sterile surgical gloves
- Lip twitch

Technique
- The procedure is performed with the limb bearing weight.
- The needle should be inserted in the palpable notch between the cranial and caudal prominences of the lateral tuberosity of the humerus (Figure 24.9).
- The needle is directed horizontally caudomedially at a 45° angle to the body.
- To penetrate the joint, the needle may need to be inserted 2 or more inches (5cm).
- A distinct "pop" may be felt as the needle penetrates the fibrous joint capsule.
- For this joint, ease of injection is not a reliable indicator of correct placement of the needle, and joint fluid often fails to flow from the needle. *Because periarticular administration of local anesthetic agent near the shoulder joint can anesthetize motor nerves, some clinicians prefer to inject a relatively short-acting, local anesthetic solution (e.g., lidocaine), to avoid prolonged paralysis of the limb, if this complication occurs. Alternatively, saline can be injected and then aspirated to determine if the needle is placed correctly, before local anesthetic solution is administered.*

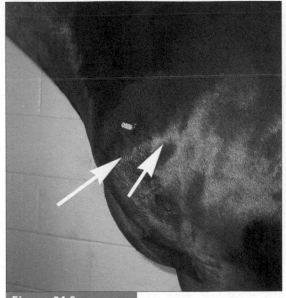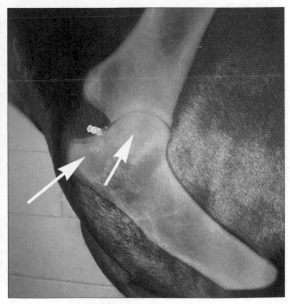

Figure 24.9 *For arthrocentesis of the scapulohumeral joint a needle is inserted in the palpable notch between the cranial and caudal prominences of the lateral tuberosity of the humerus (arrows).*

TARSAL (HOCK) JOINTS

The tarsus is composed of four principal joints, the tarsocrural, proximal intertarsal, distal inter-tarsal, and tarsometatarsal joints. The tarsocrural and proximal intertarsal joints probably communicate in all horses. The distal intertarsal and tarsometatarsal joints directly communicate in some horses, and rarely, the proximal intertarsal joint may directly communicate with the distal intertarsal, and tarsometatarsal joints. Centesis of the distal intertarsal joint for the purpose of administering local anesthetic solution or a corticosteroid for diagnosis and treatment of disease of this joint may not be necessary. After administration of mepivacaine HCL or methylprednisolone acetate in the tarsometatarsal joint, there likely is a therapeutic concentration of these drugs in the distal intertarsal joint whether or not there is direct communication of these joints.

TARSOMETATARSAL JOINT

Materials
- 20-ga, 1- or 1.5-inch needle (0.9- x 25- or 38-mm) sterile, disposable needles (some clinicians prefer a smaller gauge needle)
- 4 to 5mL local anesthetic solution if intra-articular analgesia is required
- Sterile surgical gloves
- Lip twitch

Technique
- The procedure is usually performed with the horse bearing weight on the limb. Some clinicians prefer to access the joint with the limb flexed.
- Using firm digital pressure, a small depression is palpable just proximal to the head of the fourth splint bone.
- The needle is inserted in a dorsomedial direction (Figure 24.10).
- Fluid often drips from the needle.

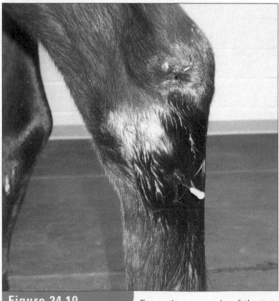
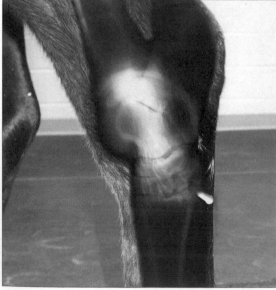

Figure 24.10 *For arthrocentesis of the tarsometatarsal joint, a needle is inserted in a dorsomedial and slightly distal direction at a small depression palpable just proximal to the head of the lateral splint bone.*

DISTAL INTERTARSAL JOINT

Materials

- 23- or 25-ga, 1-inch (0.6- or 0.5- x 25-mm) sterile, disposable needle
- 4 to 5mL local anesthetic solution if intra-articular analgesia is required
- Sterile surgical gloves
- Lip twitch

Technique

- This procedure is performed with the horse bearing weight on the limb, with the clinician positioned on the contralateral side of the horse.
- The site of centesis is found by identifying the easily palpable medial eminence of the talus. Below and caudal to this eminence is a less discernible medial eminence of the central tarsal bone. Between, and distal to these eminences, is the site for needle insertion (Figure 24.11). The needle is inserted perpendicular to the long axis of the limb, on the medial side of the tarsus in a palpable depression between the second, third, and central tarsal bones (Figure 24.12). The needle should be inserted as proximal as possible in this space to avoid entering the tarsometatarsal joint. The site may be difficult to find, especially if the joint has severe degenerative disease.
- Successful insertion of the needle into the joint can be ascertained by easy administration of drug without subcutaneous swelling, and aspiration of drug.

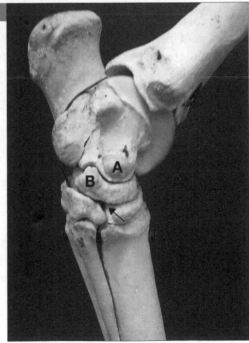

Figure 24.11

The site of centesis of the distal intertarsal joint is found by identifying the easily palpable medial eminence of the talus (A). Below and caudal to this eminence is a less discernible medial eminence of the central tarsal bone (B). Between, and distal to these eminences, is the site for needle insertion (arrow).

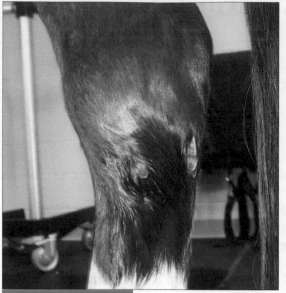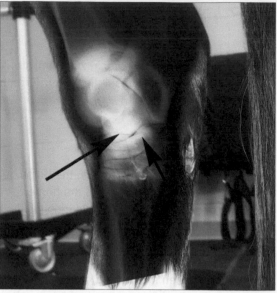

Figure 24.12 *For arthrocentesis of the distal intertarsal joint, a needle is inserted perpendicular to the long axis of the limb, on the medial side of the tarsus, in a palpable depression located midway between the dorsal and plantar surfaces of the tarsus and midway between and distal to palpable eminences (arrows) on the talus and central tarsal bones.*

TARSOCRURAL (TIBIOTARSAL) AND PROXIMAL INTERTARSAL JOINTS

The tarsocrural joint, which usually directly communicates with the proximal intertarsal joint, is the largest joint in the hock. The joint can be accessed easily via the dorsal pouch or medioplantar or lateroplantar pouches. Penetration of the medial branch of the saphenous vein (which is usually readily visible) should be avoided during centesis of the dorsal pouch.

Materials
- 20-ga, 1- or 1.5-inch (0.90- x 25- or 38-mm) sterile, disposable needle
- 10 to 20mL local anesthetic solution, if intra-articular analgesia is required
- Sterile surgical gloves
- Lip twitch

Technique
- The procedure is performed with the horse bearing weight on the limb.
- The dorsal pouch is usually palpable just distal to the medial maleolus of the tibia.
- The needle is inserted just medial or lateral to the saphenous vein, 2cm distal to the medial maleolus (Figure 24.13).
- Synovial fluid usually flows from the hub of the needle.

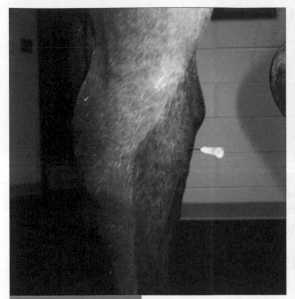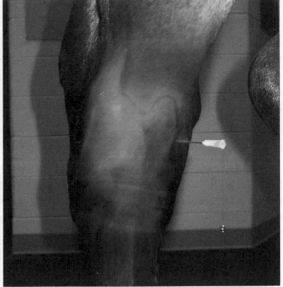

Figure 24.13 *The tarsocural joint can be accessed easily via the dorsal pouch. Penetration of the medial branch of the saphenous vein (red line) should be avoided during centesis of the dorsal pouch.*

STIFLE

The stifle is composed of three compartments, the femoropatellar joint pouch, and the medial and lateral femorotibial joint pouches. The femoropatellar joint pouch and the medial femorotibial joint pouch directly communicate in about 65% of horses, but the lateral femorotibial joint pouch seldom directly communicates with the medial compartment or with the femoropatellar joint. To rule out the stifle as a site of disease causing lameness, local anesthetic solution should be administered into each pouch. If the compartments are to be anesthetized sequentially, we prefer to first anesthetize the femoropatellar joint and then the medial compartment of the femorotibial joint.

FEMOROPATELLAR JOINT POUCH

Materials
- 20-ga, 1.5-inch (0.9- x 38-mm) sterile, disposable needle [For extremely large horses a 20-ga., 3.5-inch (8.89cm) spinal needle may be needed.]
- 30 mL local anesthetic solution if intra-articular analgesia is required
- Sterile surgical gloves
- Lip twitch

Technique
- The procedure is performed with the limb bearing weight.
- The needle is inserted caudoproximally, midway between the tibial tuberosity and the patella, between the middle and lateral patellar ligaments or between the middle and medial patellar ligaments (Figure 24.14).
- Unless the joint is distended, fluid usually is not retrieved.

MEDIAL FEMOROTIBIAL JOINT POUCH

Materials
- 20-ga, 1.5-inch (0.9- x 38-mm) sterile, disposable needle
- 20 to 30 mL local anesthetic solution if intra-articular analgesia is required
- Sterile surgical gloves
- Lip twitch

Technique
- The procedure is performed with the limb bearing weight.
- The needle is inserted perpendicular to the long axis of the limb, between the medial patellar and medial collateral ligaments just dorsal to the proximal edge of the tibia (Figure 24.14).
- Synovial fluid is usually retrieved to indicate proper needle placement.

LATERAL FEMOROTIBIAL JOINT POUCH

Materials
- 20-ga, 1.5-inch (0.9- x 38-mm) sterile, disposable needle
- 20 to 30 ml local anesthetic solution if intra-articular analgesia is required
- Sterile surgical gloves
- Lip twitch

Technique
- The procedure is performed with the horse bearing weight on the limb.
- The needle is inserted just dorsal to the proximal edge of the tibia perpendicular to the long axis of the limb just caudal to the lateral patellar ligament (Figure 24.14).
- Synovial fluid is usually retrieved, indicating proper placement of the needle.

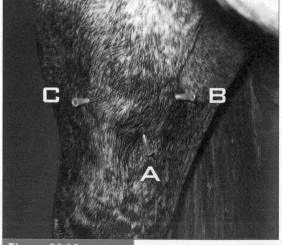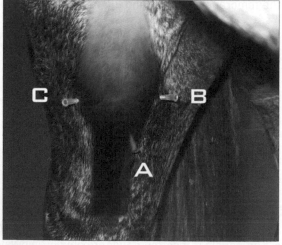

Figure 24.14 *For arthrocentesis of the femoropatellar joint (A), the needle is inserted caudoproximally, midway between the tibial tuberosity and the patella, between the middle and medial patellar ligaments (or between the middle and lateral patellar ligaments). For arthrocentesis of the medial femorotibial joint (B), the needle is inserted perpendicular to the long axis of the limb, between the medial patellar and medial collateral ligaments, just dorsal to the proximal edge of the tibia. For arthrocentesis of the lateral femorotibial joint (C), the needle is inserted just dorsal to the proximal edge of the tibia perpendicular to the long axis of the limb caudal to the lateral patellar ligament.*

COXOFEMORAL (HIP) JOINT

The hip joint is difficult to enter, and with improper needle placement, the sciatic nerve can be damaged.

Materials
- 25-ga (0.5-mm) needle and several mLs local anesthetic solution to inject subcutaneously at the site of needle placement (optional)
- 18-ga, 6-inch (1.2-mm- x 15-cm) spinal needle. A longer needle is necessary to reach the joint in heavily muscled horses.
- 20 to 30 mL local anesthetic solution if intra-articular analgesia is required
- Sterile surgical gloves
- Lip twitch

Technique
- The procedure is performed with the limb bearing weight.
- The site of needle placement is the middle of the shelf of the anterior trochanter major. This site is difficult to palpate in most horses. It can be found by first identifying the more easily palpated posterior trochanter major. The anterior trochanter major is found about 2.5 inches (5 cm) ventral and cranial to this eminence.
- Local anesthetic solution is administered subcutaneously.
- The needle is inserted just dorsal to the middle of the shelf of the anterior trochanter major (Figure 24.15). The needle is directed horizontal to the ground in a slightly cranial direction (Figure 24.16).
- The joint is entered after inserting nearly the entire shaft of the needle.
- Synovial fluid can occasionally be aspirated. Aspiration of local anesthetic solution after administration indicates proper needle placement.

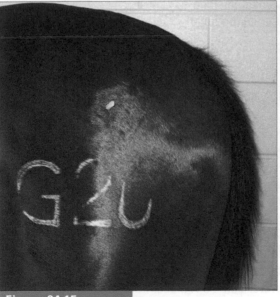 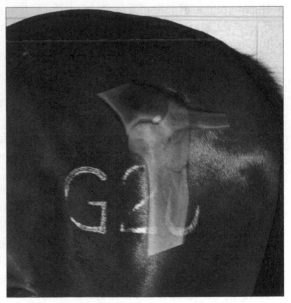

Figure 24.15 *For arthrocentesis of the coxofemoral joint, an 18-ga, 6-inch (1.2- x 15-cm) spinal needle is inserted horizontal to the ground in a slightly cranial direction, just dorsal to the middle of the shelf of the anterior trochanter major.*

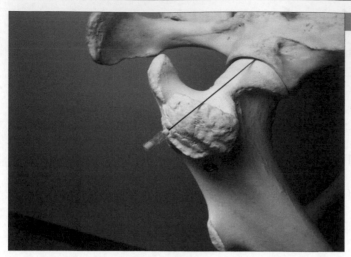

Figure 24.16

For arthrocentesis of the coxofemoral joint, the needle is directed slightly cranially in a horizontal plane.

CENTESIS OF THE NAVICULAR BURSA

Five different techniques for centesis of the navicular bursa have been described. The following technique was shown to be the most accurate.

Materials
- 25-ga (0.5-mm) needle and 0.5 - 1 mL local anesthetic solution to inject subcutaneously at the site of needle placement
- 20-ga, 3.5-inch (1.1- x 8.89-cm) spinal needle
- 2 to 3 mL local anesthetic solution if intra-bursal analgesia is required
- Sterile surgical gloves
- Lip twitch
- Sedation (optional)
- Hickman block (optional) to stabilize the foot in a flexed position
- 0.5 – 1 mL sterile, water-soluble, radiocontrast material (optional)
- Radiographic equipment (optional)

Technique
- The skin between the bulbs of the heel, immediately above the coronary band, is desensitized with 0.5 to 1mL of local anesthetic solution.
- The foot is marked halfway between the most dorsal and the most palmar aspect of the coronary band and 1cm distal to the coronary band. This spot marks the site of the long axis of the navicular bone.
- The spinal needle is advanced toward the bisecting point between the sagittal plane of the foot and the long axis of the navicular bone (i.e., angled and advanced sagittally toward the mark on the hoof wall) (Figure 24.17).
- The spinal needle is advanced until the tip of the needle contacts bone and the stylet is removed for administration of drug. The tip of the needle is determined to be within the navicular bursa by low resistance to injection and the ability to aspirate the injected contents of the syringe.
- To verify centesis of the bursa, 0.5 – 1mL sterile, water-soluble radiocontrast solution can be administered along with the drug. On a laterally projected radiograph taken immediately after administration of contrast solution, the bursa appears as a comma shaped structure surrounding the caudal portion of the navicular bone (Figure 24.18).

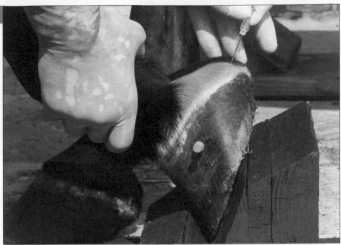

Figure 24.17

For centesis of the navicular bursa, the spinal needle is angled and advanced sagittally toward a mark on the hoof wall halfway between the most dorsal and the most palmar aspect of the coronary band and 1cm distal to the coronary band.

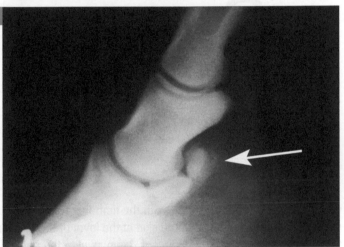

Figure 24.18

To verify centesis of the navicular bursa, 0.5 – 1mL sterile, water-soluble radiocontrast solution can be administered along with the drug. On a laterally projected radiograph taken immediately after administration of contrast solution, the bursa appears as a comma shaped structure (arrow) surrounding the caudal portion of the navicular bone.

CENTESIS OF THE DIGITAL FLEXOR TENDON SHEATH

Centesis of the pouches (Figure 24.19) of the deep digital flexor tendon sheath is difficult when the sheath is not distended with synovial fluid. An approach through the palmar annular ligament of the fetlock (palmar axial sesamoidean approach) was found to be reliable for consistent synoviocentesis of the digital flexor tendon sheath. The palmar axial sesamoidean approach is less likely to result in synovial hemorrhage than other approaches.

Materials
- 20- ga, 1.5 inch (0.90 x 38 mm) sterile, disposable needle
- 10 to 15mL local anesthetic solution if intra-synovial analgesia is required
- Sterile surgical gloves
- Lip twitch

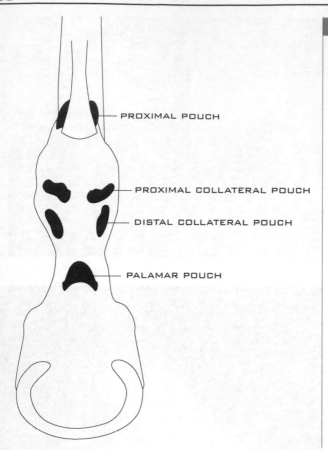

— PROXIMAL POUCH

— PROXIMAL COLLATERAL POUCH

— DISTAL COLLATERAL POUCH

— PALAMAR POUCH

Figure 24.19

Pouches of the deep digital flexor tendon sheath are shown in this diagram.

Technique

- The procedure is performed with the limb flexed.
- The needle placed through the skin at the level of the midbody of the lateral proximal sesamoid bone, through the palmar annular ligament, 3 mm axial to the palpable palmar border of the lateral proximal sesamoid bone and immediately palmar to the palmar digital neurovascular bundle (Figure 24.20).
- The needle is inserted in a transverse plane and advanced at an angle to the sagittal plane, aiming toward the central intersesamoidean region to a depth of 1.5 to 2.0 cm.

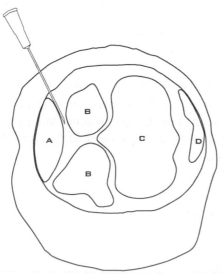

Figure 24.20

For centesis of the deep digital flexor tendon sheath, the needle is inserted in a transverse plane and advanced at an angle to the sagittal plane, aiming toward the central intersesamoidean region to a depth of 1.5 to 2.0 cm. In this cross section through the proximal sesamoid bones, A = flexor tendons, B = proximal sesamoid bones, C = metacarpus / metatarsus and D = extensor tendon.

CENTESIS OF A CERVICAL FACET JOINT

Centesis of a cervical facet joint is performed in horses with signs of neck pain, and radiographic, ultrasonographic or scintigraphic evidence of disease of a facet joint. Centesis is usually performed for administration of local anesthetic solution or a corticosteroid. Lesions are most commonly found in the joints of facets joining cervical vertebrae 5 & 6 and 6 & 7. Different approaches to these joints are described, but all techniques rely on ultrasonic guidance.

Materials
- Ultrasonographic equipment with a 5 or 7.5 MHz sector or linear transducer
- 25-ga (0.5-mm) needle and local anesthetic solution
- A sedative such as xylazine or detomidine
- A 20- or 18-ga, 3.5-in (0.90 or 1.2-mm, 8.89-cm), spinal needle
- Because the procedure is usually performed for horses suspected to have arthritis of facet joints, intra-articular medication such as a corticosteroid may be administered.

Technique
- The site of cervical facet arthropathy is identified using diagnostic imaging.
- For the average sized horse, the width of a cervical vertebra is the width of a hand palm (Figure 24.21). The approximate site of centesis is found by placing hand over hand from the poll along the cervical spine, each hand covering the width of a cervical vertebra. The transverse processes of the cervical vertebrae are palpable and the facet joint is located above the caudal extent (dorsal tubercule) of the transverse process (Figure 24.22).
- The region of the site of centesis is surgically prepared.
- The joint between two adjacent articular facets is identified ultrasonograhically in the center of the imaging field, using a probe that has been surgically scrubbed or placed in a sterile surgical glove filled with coupling gel. The skin should be liberally soaked with isopropyl alcohol to achieve acoustic coupling.
- With the ultrasound probe in place, the site of centesis just above the probe is again surgically prepared and local anesthetic solution is administered subcutaneously.

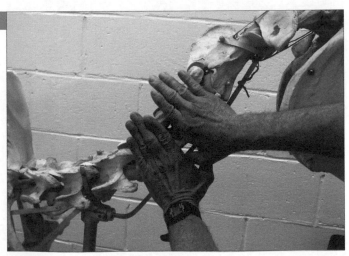

Figure 24.21

For the average sized horse, the width of a cervical vertebra is the width of a hand palm. The approximate site of centesis is found by placing hand over hand from the poll along the cervical spine, each hand covering the width of a cervical vertebra.

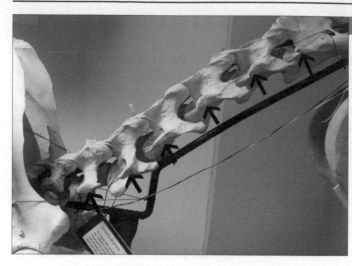

Figure 24.22

The transverse processes (arrows) of the cervical vertebrae are palpable and the facet joint is located above the caudal extent (dorsal tubercle) of the transverse process. A 20 ga needle has been inserted into the vertebral joint C5-6.

- The spinal needle is inserted just dorsal to the ultrasound probe and advanced at an angle (about 30-45°) that will aim it at the approximate site of the joint (Figure 24.23). The joint space can be widened if the horse's neck is flexed away from the site of centesis.
- Using ultrasonic guidance, the needle is directed into (or at least close to) the joint space (Figure 24.24) and drug is injected.
- Joint fluid can often be aspirated if the needle is placed correctly. If the needle is within the joint, drug cannot be visualized ultrasonographically as it is administered.

Complications
- The needle cannot be placed in some joints with advanced arthropathy. Periarticular administration of corticosteroid, however, may be beneficial.

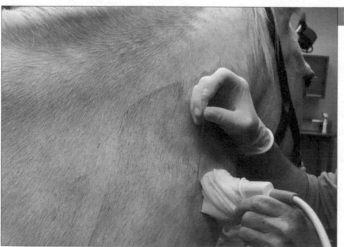

Figure 24.23

For centesis of a cervical facet joint, a 20-ga, 3.5-in (0.9-mm, 8.89-cm), spinal needle is inserted and advanced at an angle that will aim it at the approximate site of the joint which is identified using ultrasonography.

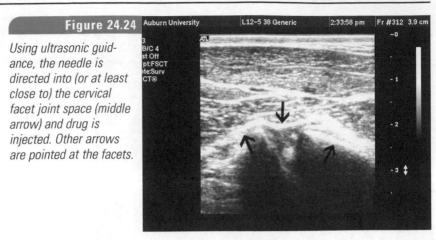

Figure 24.24

Using ultrasonic guidance, the needle is directed into (or at least close to) the cervical facet joint space (middle arrow) and drug is injected. Other arrows are pointed at the facets.

CENTESIS OF THE TEMPOROMANDIBULAR (TM) JOINT

The TM joint in the horse has rarely been mentioned as problematic, however, with recent advancements in equine dentistry and geriatric medicine we are finding that the TM joint may develop the same diseases, as do other joints in the horse. Centesis of the TM joint is made through a caudodorsal approach.

Materials
- 20- ga, 1.5 inch (0.90 x 38 mm) sterile disposable needles
- 5mL local anesthetic solution if intra-articular analgesia is required
- Sedative
- Sterile gloves
- Lip twitch
- An assistant facilitates the procedure by controlling the position of the head as well as manipulating the mandible in order to palpate the joint.

Technique
- The procedure is performed on a sedated horse.
- The lateral margin of the mandibular condyle is identified approximately midway on a line between the lateral canthus of the eye and the base of the ear (Figure 24.25). Its location can be confirmed by palpation while manipulating the mandible from side to side.
- Locate a soft depression 1-2 cm dorsal and 1 cm caudal to the condyle.
- The needle is inserted in this soft depression in a rostral ventral direction to a depth of approximately 1 inch (25 mm) (Figure 24.26).
- Fluid may fill the needle hub. If the needle hits bone, the needle should be partially withdrawn and directed more ventrally. If the needle is directed too far ventrally, it may become embedded in the articular disc and should be partially withdrawn.

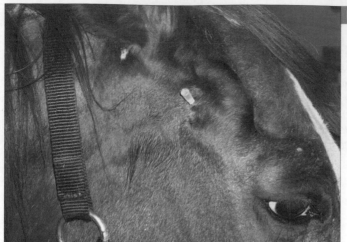

Figure 24.25

The lateral margin of the mandibular condyle is identified on a line approximately midway between the lateral canthus of the eye and the base of the ear.

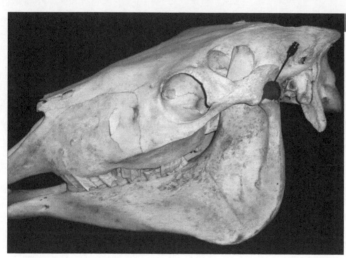

Figure 24.26

For centesis of the temporomandibular joint, a 20-ga, 1.5 in needle is inserted in a rostral ventral direction to a depth of approximately 1 inch in a soft depression 1-2 cm dorsal and 1 cm caudal to the mandibular condyle.

SUGGESTED READINGS

de Mercado RV, Stover SM. Comparison of six techniques for a lateral approach to the coffin joint. *44th Annual Proceedings American Association of Equine Practitioners,* December 6-9, 1998, Baltimore, MD 178-179.

Grisel GR, Grant BD, Rantanen NW. Arthrocentesis of the equine cervical facets. *42nd Annual Proceedings American Association of Equine Practitioners,* December 8-11, 1996, Denver, CO. 197-198.

Hassel DM, Stover SM, Yarbrough TB, Drake CM, Taylor KT. Palmar-plantar axial sesamoidean approach to the digital flexor tendon sheath in horses, *J Am Vet Med Assoc* 217:1343, 2000.

Lewis RD. Techniques for arthrocentesis of equine shoulder, elbow stifle and hip joints. *42nd Annual Proceedings American Association of Equine Practitioners,* December 8-11, 1996, Denver, CO. 55-63.

May KA, Moll HD, Howard RD, Pleasant RS, Gregg JM. Arthroscopic anatomy of the equine temporomandibular joint. *Veterinary Surgery* 30:564-571, 2001.

Misheff M, Stover SM. Comparison of two techniques for arthrocentesis of the equine metacarpophalangeal joint. *Equine Veterinary Journal* 23:273-276, 1991.

Moyer W, Carter GK. Techniques to facilitate intra-articular injection of equine joints. *42nd Annual Proceedings American Association of Equine Practitioners,* December 8-11, 1996, Denver, CO. 48-54.

Schramme MC, Boswell JC, Hamhoughias K, Toulson K, Viitanen M. An *in vitro* study to compare 5 different techniques for injection of the navicular bursa in the horse, *Equine Vet J* 32:263, 2000.

Schumacher John, Schramme MC, Schumacher Jim, DeGraves F, Smith RKW, Coker M. A review of recent studies concerning diagnostic analgesia of the equine forefoot. *49th Annual Proceedings American Association of Equine Practitioners,* November 21-25, 2003, New Orleans, LA. 312-316.

INDEX

T - #0683 - 101024 - C0 - 254/178/6 - PB - 9781893441996 - Gloss Lamination